THE SILENT PASSAGE

Gail Sheehy is the author of ten books, including her landmark work, *Passages*. In a 1991 survey of the books that have most influenced people's lives, *Passages* was listed in the top ten.

Ms Sheehy was one of the original contributors to *New York* magazine and is now a contributing editor of *Vanity Fair*. She is the mother of two daughters and lives in New York City with her husband, publisher and editor Clay Felker.

GAIL SHEEHY

The Silent Passage
Menopause

HarperCollins*Publishers*

HarperCollins*Publishers*
77–85 Fulham Palace Road,
Hammersmith, London W6 8JB

This paperback edition 1994
1   3   5   7   9   8   6   4   2

First published in Great Britain by
HarperCollins*Publishers* 1993

Copyright © G. Merritt Corporation 1991, 1992, 1993

The Author asserts the moral right to
be identified as the author of this work

ISBN 0 00 637967 2

Set in Walbaum

Printed in Great Britain by
HarperCollinsManufacturing Glasgow

Contents

⊃⊲

'The Need to Know and the Fear of Knowing'

The Perimenopause Panic

The Menopause Gateway

Coalescence

Author's Note

A word on method. In my earlier American research, I sought out women from all social levels and races and regions of the United States. I conducted intimate group interviews, as well as collected individual life histories, in places as dissimilar as Eugene, Oregon; Rochester, New York; Louisville, Kentucky; downtown Los Angeles and Beverly Hills in California; Queens and Manhattan in New York. Participants included privileged women and low income government workers, women of colour and polite white suburbanites, mid-forties women anticipating the Change and women in their sixties who could look back on it with some perspective. In my American research, I interviewed over a hundred women in various stages of menopause.

More detailed medical information was also necessary to raise awareness among women as health consumers. In my research I freely crossed disciplines, reaching beyond the obvious medical practitioners – gynaecologists, breast surgeons and internists – to endocrinologists who study the hard science of hormones, and epidemiologists who measure all the factors contributing to a condition like menopause in large populations. Additional light was shed on this complex life transition by interviews with research physiologists, neuroscientists, psychologists, psychiatrists and gerontologists; and practical approaches to coping with it were suggested by nutritional and Chinese medicine doctors. For a larger historical and evolutionary perspective I consulted scholars in sociology and anthropology, historians and primate researchers. I interviewed a total of ninety experts.

I was not altogether alone in my explorations. Patricia Allen, an obstetrician-gynaecologist in private practice in Manhattan and on the staff at New York Hospital, took an interest in my efforts – both as my personal doctor and as a professional committed to expanding health education for women. Dr Allen introduced me to top specialists in related fields, and took to the trenches with me to listen in on some of the group interviews in other parts of the country. It was a journey of discovery that helped me, as the cultural translator, to shed stereotypes and orthodoxies.

My thanks go to Dr William J. Ledger, professor and chairman of Obstetrics and Gynecology at New York Hospital-Cornell Medical Center, and to Dr Robert Lindsay, a leading research endocrinologist in the field of menopause medicine and practitioner at Helen Hayes Bone Center, both of whom read the manuscript and added suggestions and refinements. In Britain, Dr Malcolm Whitehead, director of the Menopause Clinic of Kings College Hospital, London, and president of the International Menopause Society, together with his senior research fellow, Dr Mike Ellerington, were mines of information on the state of research and treatment in the UK. Dr John Moran, a private gynaecologist at the Hormonal Health Care Centre on Harley Street, was very helpful in sharing his experience of treating thousands of women over the course of fifteen years in menopause clinics. Dr Shyam Singha, a world-renowned homeopathic practitioner and teacher, added a non-traditional treatment perspective.

It has been my privilege to work on this edition with one of Britain's most distinguished editors, Michael Fishwick, and my good fortune to have the assistance of Juliet Van Oss.

The women who gallantly contributed their personal stories to this book are also my partners. Some of their names and backgrounds had to be altered, but others offered their real names. To each one I offer thanks for striking one more small blow for normalization of a proud stage of life.

Introduction

This book has two wellsprings. The first was my own ignorance. About pregnancy we are taught everything one could want to know. I remember finding books on natural childbirth in the library and teaching myself the breathing exercises, so that by the time I went into labour I felt fully prepared. By contrast, I went into menopause knowing nothing – not even that I was in it. Like so many women who have always enjoyed good health and who prided myself, upon reaching my mid-forties, on having achieved a fair degree of control over my life, I was sure I would just 'sail right through it'. Instead, I veered off course, lost some of the wind in my sails, and almost capsized.

But in trying to learn or talk about menopause, I found myself up against a powerful and mysterious taboo. My friends were adrift in the same fog of inexcusable ignorance. We couldn't help one another because none of us knew enough. Or we didn't want to know. I remember having to stifle a gasp as I sat in the kitchen of a friend who insisted, 'Oh, it doesn't apply to me' – with her bottle of oestrogen tablets staring us in the face! Scarcely anyone seemed to be willing to talk to me honestly about the Change of Life. The subject was a real room emptier. The second wellspring of this book, then, became an intention to break the silence.

Putting on my investigative journalist's hat, I explored the state of knowledge on menopause in America, Canada, and Europe and discovered an appalling state of ignorance about a transition that half the population of the world faces. After some thought, I decided to break the silence and go public with my own, not uncommon experience and eventually found other well-known women willing to do the same. Initially, Tina Brown took the bold step of publishing my material in *Vanity Fair*. The electrifying response to that article was the impetus to expand my research and interviews into a book.

Who would have dreamed a book about menopause would become a best-seller? When *The Silent Passage* was first published in America in May, 1992, it touched a nerve much deeper than I had imagined. I knew from my explorations how backward we are in basic scientific research on a condition that goes back to prehistory. Menopause is not some new environmental toxin, after all, yet as the director of the US National Institutes of Health, Dr Bernadine Healy, sums it up, 'It's disgraceful that in our sophisticated world of medicine, with our phenomenal track record, we still can't answer simple questions about menopause.' But I had no concept of the shocking breadth of ignorance and denial women would discover among themselves. Nor did they.

It is as though there were a conspiracy of silence which has hidden the fact of how much power older women potentially wield. And guess who's at the heart of the conspiracy? We are.

As I travelled around the United States giving lectures and appearing on TV and radio talk shows, the conversation about menopause had to be started up from scratch in each city. The effort was tantamount to breaking the ice at a particularly stiff cocktail party, the kind where everyone knows the host has just lost his job or his wife is having it off with the caterer but nobody mentions it. Reactions from male talk show hosts were sometimes comical.

'Menopause,' gulped a Cleveland man on the midday news. 'Is that like – impotence?'

'Um, no,' I murmured lamely. Only later did I think of the right comeback:

'Baldness. Is that like – Alzheimer's?'

When I appeared on the 'Oprah Winfrey Show', her producer admitted on the air that they had had an easier time booking guests to talk about murdering their spouses than about menopause. Six months after the conversation opened in the United States, menopause had become one of the hottest topics in the media, bookstores, and on the lecture circuit, as a new generation of women brought to it a bold new attitude. The safety in numbers was exhilarating to all of us. The silence, at last, was being broken.

While menopause itself is part of what it is to be a woman, the menopausal experience is coloured by culture. Even within Western cultures as similar as the United States and Great Britain, I have often been struck by the very different attitudes towards subjects such as successful women, ageing, diet, exercise, and so on, and suspected it would be the same with menopause. It is.

My curiosity about the impact of culture plunged me into cross-cultural research for this new edition of the book, using Great Britain as the comparative culture. Certain differences were to be expected. A state-run medical system, as opposed to a private one, strongly conditions the way women and their doctors treat a matter that is not considered a serious health problem. And like other European countries, Britain has a wider spectrum of drugs and more acceptance of non-traditional practices for handling menopause than the United States. But the more intriguing comparisons, I found, were in subjective attitudes about this passage, and the whole subject of ageing that it inevitably stirs up.

British women are, on the whole, better informed than American women about hormone replacement therapy (HRT). The media in Britain and Europe have given considerable attention to the pros and cons of hormones over the past five years. But outside that narrow consideration, I found, many women put blinkers on and refuse to acknowledge the deeper psychosexual questions and long-term health questions raised by this transition.

'My response to the word menopause is so overlaid with doom, which it shouldn't be,' mused Fay Weldon, the novelist famed for her witty send-ups of male sexual vanity. 'To define yourself as menopausal is, in a way, a mistake,' she decided in the course of a lengthy interview. 'It's a word used by men to define the cause of your being horrible, miserable and unattractive, as they see it. If women embrace this as a term, they're inviting a definition which is diminishing to them. Hormone levels are not the total sum of a human being: there is more to their misery than that.'

In her words I heard a common discomfort about committing oneself to the existence of such a problematic passage. The popular British novelist now living in America, Barbara Taylor Bradford, put up an even more defiant resistance. Remembering as a girl how her aunts in England had talked about the Change in hushed, somewhat ominous tones, she simply vowed to herself when she hit fifty, 'To hell with that. I'm not going to pay any attention. It's not going to have any effect on me!'

One might characterize this common British attitude: *If I don't acknowledge it, it doesn't exist.* The same attitude was put slightly differently by Eve Pollard, the normally outspoken editor of the *Sunday Express*: 'If you don't talk about it, you might just float through it.' She acknowledges, however, 'We certainly share the American nervousness about getting older.'

After intensive interviewing in the United Kingdom, I began to sense that the subject of menopause has been reduced almost entirely to a debate about hormone replacement and has become polarized around two opposing views. One view holds that HRT is the elixir of life. It is promoted by the bottom feeders among the tabloids with desperately shrill headlines like, MY SEX LIFE IS TERRIFIC BECAUSE I'M ON HRT! Rich, glamorous, famous women like Joan Collins and Kate O'Mara praise hormone treatment to the skies, claiming it keeps them young and sexy.

'When you're my age, you must go on HRT,' the lusty O'Mara proselytyzes younger actresses. 'It's wonderful, it's brilliant, it's the last great frontier to women's true emancipation. The contraceptive pill was the first great step, and hormone replacement therapy is the second great one.' The actress doesn't mind at all disclosing her age: fifty-three. As she told me, that's the whole point.

The opposite view defies the 'medicalization of menopause', and holds that it is a natural process; one should not interfere with nature. All the fuss is put down to a futile vanity. I found a whole arc of subtle distinctions within this perspective. Dorothy Rowe, a sage British psychologist in her sixties who writes and gardens in Sheffield, represents the sensible-shoes outlook.

'In Britain, there simply isn't this feeling that you have to stay young. Cher and Joan Collins are not role models here. The Queen is a role model. A lot of women dress like her. Sensible, not flashy.'

Eve Pollard expressed the different perspective of a younger, more combative generation: 'Sharing the Queen's attitude is fine and good *only* if you're upper class. If you are just out there watching Woody Allen going for 21-year-olds, you know which way this thing goes.'

The extreme version of the 'natural menopause' view is represented by Germaine Greer's brilliant polemic, *The Change*. Rummaging through historical accounts of the ageing female, Greer rails against the negative projections, but in defiance seems to embrace them. She writes about the invisibility of the middle-aged woman and of feeling tired, disillusioned, and finished at fifty. '. . . Convincing yourself you're happy and fulfilled may be deluding yourself to the point of insanity,' she says. The silver lining she finds in her unwanted liberation is 'to be relieved from passion'. She counsels women to resort to behaving like crones as the way to register their visibility. 'You're expected to be dreadful. So you might as well act it.' Making a talisman of her own frustrating experience with hormone replacement therapy, Greer properly faults the medical establishment for conspiring to make women dependent on pills and patches that have been woefully undertested. But her bitter manifesto serves also to blind women to the renewal of energy, new passions and purposes possible at this time of life.

What is lost in the bombardment of these opposing views

is the main point: that we are living longer lives than ever before. Since there has been virtually no period in the history of the human species when evolution has favoured post-menopausal females, we shall have to favour ourselves. We shall *have to* intervene – medically, hormonally, psychologically, spiritually – because we cannot assume that ageing will go smoothly. Evolution didn't provide for it. But my impression from talking to thousands of women all over America and Europe is that this new perspective – only milliseconds old in evolutionary terms – has not caught up with most people.

The middle classes in Britain may believe they are well-informed; observers such as Fay Weldon are sceptical: 'They'd on the whole rather not know – for if we don't know it doesn't matter.'

But it does matter. It matters whether or not a woman in her sixties finds it painful to walk or even bend as a result of osteoporosis. It matters when a woman in her fifties has a heart attack. It matters that women look these possibilities in the eye, because the way in which they approach menopause will affect their risk of suffering from these diseases. Naturally, parts of our bodies are going to break down with the ageing process. Since we can expect to live to our eighties – whether we wish to or not – do we want to have three parts shut down and one part still going?

To most Britons, expectations of life beyond age fifty are still based on outdated stereotypes of an older generation. The retirement age for women is still sixty. Many approach retirement with the attitude, 'I've had a long, hard life, and retirement is the rest I deserve.' They seem to accept, along with Germaine Greer, that 'the climacteric is the antechamber of death'.

In fact, death for the average fifty-year-old British woman is more than thirty years away. Who wants to rest for thirty years? Even if you want to, that much rest is hazardous to your health.

Startling realities about being over fifty in the United Kingdom come out of recent comprehensive reports done for the

Carnegie Inquiry into the Third Age. The Third Age is defined as people aged fifty to seventy-five, and we will be hearing more and more from them. At present, the UK has fourteen million Third Agers. By the year 2020, people aged fifty to seventy-five will represent the *largest* population group in the culture.

The same age group will also dominate American culture: ninety-three million people will be fifty to seventy-five; and with those over seventy-five added on, the total will be a stunning 114 million people out of a projected US population of 327 million by the year 2020. (80 million will be between thirty and forty-nine; 60 million between sixteen and twenty-nine, and 72 million under sixteen.) Supporting research for the Third Age Inquiry suggests that there is broad agreement among the middle classes (less among the working classes) that older people should live a much more active life in the future. But outmoded attitudes still obtain.

People say they are waiting for retirement to do all the things they've always wanted to do. When they actually get there, the only two things they do more of are reading the newspaper and watching television. Unpaid volunteer work and participation in active leisure pursuits actually fall off after people retire. For one thing, they lose links with the larger world that used to exist through the workplace or their children's schools. Moreover, as industry continues to use early retirement as a way of de-manning, people are encouraged to take an attractive lump-sum redundancy payment. It's lovely for a while, but then it's gone. Basic necessities for mobility and mental stimulation, like a car or the fare to travel, become an unaffordable luxury.

For women in the Third Age, the problem is first and foremost financial. Marriages in Britain are breaking up at a much later age. The proportion of postmenopausal women who can expect to be divorced will rise from 3 percent to 15 percent by the year 2020. The study director, Terry Banks, warns: 'An enormous number of those women will face poverty.'

*

In the end, it's not so much what happens to us in life that matters, but how we interpret what happens to us. Every woman over fifty must wrestle, to some degree, with feeling like a discard. A large number of British women arrive at this stage with very little self-confidence, according to Rowe. 'They've been taught that they must always deprecate themselves. They think that nobody wants them, and because women live so long, that becomes a central problem of their old age.' In addition, 'any woman who has to live on the basic old age pension here, without family to make her life better, really has a struggle,' says Rowe. 'An enormous amount of her energy has to go into simply making ends meet.'

Any one of these daunting sociological realities is made more likely insurmountable if a woman has not consciously maintained her health over the menopausal transition. Teresa Gorman MP, the oldest woman ever elected to British Parliament, asserts that 'a third of the hospital beds in Britain, and presumably the same in Australia, are occupied by women who have some problem related to untreated menopause'.

By contrast, a woman who has provided for her health and salted away her own employment pension, and who believes, at sixty, that she *deserves* a full and interesting life, will probably have cultivated many different skills and great and small passions. She very likely has goals and dreams that will, by intention, outlast her life span.

Menopause must be approached today with a different attitude, one that is self-valuing, rather than self-deprecating. Making the effort to change eating, smoking, sleeping and exercise habits, and taking the time to experiment with hormone replacement or homeopathic practices to help rebalance the body around its new hormonal state, is not an issue of vanity, or attracting men, or succumbing to Western culture's preoccupation with youth. It is an issue of physical and mental *health*. Yet general practitioners in the UK are not pressed to treat menopause seriously, and too many avoid it. There are, however, strong voices among British women in public life who are demonstrating the savvy and self-confidence and startling energy that are the most notable characteristics of the contemporary menopausal woman. Some of them have already broken the silence about menopause on the floor of Parliament.

'We are the pioneers,' asserted the indefatigable MP Edwina Currie when I talked to her. 'It's the first time ever that women have risen to quite high levels in public life. Speaking out in books like this is important, because we are sharing our secrets with millions of women who otherwise might be writing themselves off.'

Menopause is like a thumbprint – it is that individual. Each woman will have to decide for herself whether or not the benefits of hormone therapy are worth the risks in her case, and at what point she will give up the fight to remain the young woman she was and accept her future self. The important point is that women in the Change today have choices; they need not follow anybody's manifesto. This book is meant to empower women by informing them of the many different ways they can protect their bodies and promote their mental wellbeing through menopause and beyond, so they can look forward to finding passion and purpose apart from being a vessel of reproduction.

Some of the stories herein are cautionary tales of embittered or self-deluding women. And some are snapshots of women who have given themselves every chance to live out the length of their days. I hope the stories of the women in this book will act as a catalyst for honest conversations about the menopausal experience between mothers and daughters, wives and husbands, women and their doctors.

This book, then, has three purposes: first, to shatter the myths about menopause. Second, to emphasize that menopause is a health issue, and to prompt women on how to educate their doctors and the men in their lives. And finally, most important, I want to leave readers with another way to think about this stage of a woman's life – what I call the Second Adulthood.

I am happy to report that in only the first year since publication of this book in America, a new camaraderie is developing among women who are full of juice, humour, and determination to turn this passage into a celebration. They are forming 'fan clubs' to share experiences and swap tips and develop directories of doctors who are knowledgeable or at least educable about menopause. In many ways, there has never been a better time in history to pass through menopause. In that spirit, California women asked me to pass along this motto, which they are hanging up on their office walls:

WOMEN DON'T HAVE HOT FLUSHES
THEY HAVE POWER SURGES!

G.S.

'The Need to Know
and the
Fear of Knowing'

A group of recognizably high-powered media women on the shady side of forty were spaced around the table between their husbands and lovers at a Washington dinner party when a single sentence shattered their well-groomed calm. It came out of the mouth of the stunning network newswoman who ordinarily speaks in ninety-second bursts of inside-the-Beltway shorthand.

'Okay, there are only two subjects worth talking about – menopause and face lifts.' It was as though a nine-hundred-pound gorilla had just jumped up on the table.

We think of ourselves as so liberated today we can talk about anything. People will tell strangers about their abortions or alcoholism, even declare on national television that they are HIV positive with the AIDS virus; yet women still shrink from mentioning, even to their good women friends, the fear they might be menopausal. And just let a man suggest to his sleepless, perspiry, weepy wife that her uncharacteristic moods and symptoms might have something to do with menopause; he's bound to get a blanket denial: 'What are you talking about! I'm too young!'

Menopause may be the last taboo. The first friend to whom I mentioned the subject is a sultry-looking woman of fifty (pre-baby boom). She has always prided herself on her appearance and gained much of her status from creatively supporting her husband, a successful author who looks somewhat younger than she. I asked if she had ever talked with anyone about menopause.

'No. And I don't want to.'

'Women don't bring up the subject around you?'

'One friend did,' she said sourly. 'I haven't seen her since.'

Another friend, a public television producer whose natural temperament is appallingly calm, recalled with rueful laughter her first sign of the Change of Life. She was seated between two titans of industry at a high-protocol Park Avenue dinner party, the kind where the place cards look like tracings from the *Book of Kells*, and she was feeling particularly confident and pretty in her new black designer suit with its flattering white satin collar when out of the blue a droplet of something hit her collar. Then another drop. What the – was the help dribbling wine? Could there be a leaky ceiling under all that gorgeous boiserie? Suddenly she noticed her husband's gaze turn to alarm from across the table: What horrible thing was happening to her? She put a hand to her face. Her forehead was wet as a swamp.

Oh no, said her eyes, *not me!*, as the moisture began running in rivulets down her face and slipping off her chin – *plop* – on to her pearly satin collar. Should I pick up the white linen napkin and wipe my forehead? She reached for the 500-threads-per-inch napery, hesitated – *No, all the makeup will come off on the damn napkin* – when a few more plops fell into her decolletage. Frantic, she began dabbing at her face. Trying to pretend it wasn't happening, she turned to her dinner partner and began smiling and mopping, chatting and fanning, laughing at his jokes and dabbing, trying to keep up her end of the conversation, while she wanted nothing more in this world than to disappear into the kitchen and tear off her clothes and open the freezer door – never mind that it was February – and just *stand there*.

That was a year ago. She and her husband have had the Thermostat Wars usual in menopausal households – 'It's freezing in here!' 'No, it's boiling.' 'Did you turn the thermostat below fifty again?' 'Oh, why don't you just get some flannel pajamas!' But the producer is one of the lucky ones: she has had no other indicators beyond hot flushes that she is passing into another stage of life.

It happens to every woman. Pregnancy we can choose to go through or not. With menopause there is no choice. It happens to teachers and discount store clerks and dental hygienists, who nonetheless have to function in public, on their feet, every day. It happens to Navy pilots and grey-haired graduate students and former Olympic athletes, who are accustomed to demanding the highest physical and mental performance from themselves. It happens to women of colour, to women in the home, to women of glamour like Kate O'Mara.

O'Mara was in Hollywood filming a segment for *Dynasty*, where she played Joan Collins' younger sister, when the biological clock suddenly clanged. She was forty-six or -seven, and her TV persona as a slim-hipped she-cat (who also happens to be a serious Shakespearean actress) was very well preserved. The director told O'Mara to sit in a bubble bath while she spoke her lines over a telephone.

Dear God, this bath is hot, she thought. Could the prop girl splash some cold water in it? It must be the California climate, she consoled herself. More cold water, please! But it wasn't the water. It was, inescapably, drenchingly, and most unsexily, a hot flush. O'Mara leapt from the bath and thought, 'That's it. It's all over.'

Since that incident five years ago, the volatile actress has discovered hormone replacement therapy and become a total devotee. Her publicity photos today present a bust-thrusting sex siren propped on stiletto heels with a plume of streaked brown hair, a performer who obviously takes considerable care in the attempt to freeze time. Because she doesn't conform to society's outdated notions of how a woman in her fifties *should* look, the tabloids often ridicule her: 'At an age when most women should be sitting in their rocking chairs knitting little garments for their grandchildren, Ms O'Mara is seen flaunting herself in a miniskirt and dancing with a man twenty years younger than herself.' Feminists attack her for doing all this only to look attractive to men. O'Mara, divorced for the last eighteen years, huffily denies the charge.

'What they don't understand is the longer my looks and my energy last, the longer my career lasts. It's about looking and feeling energetic. It doesn't matter whether you ever want to see a man in your bed again.'

Raquel and Farrah, Liz and Ann-Margret, too, must deal with menopause. These Hollywood icons are hardly over the hill. In fact, they are hitting a new stride.

But they never mention the big M.

The longer we keep menopause in the closet or pretend it's nothing to get excited about, the longer we perpetuate the ignorance and veil of myths surrounding it. The central myth is that menopause is a time in a woman's life when she goes batty for a few years – subject to wild rages and deep depressions – and after it she mourns her lost youth and fades into the woodwork. In truth, menopause is a bridge to the most vital and liberated period in a woman's life. Certainly hormones have a powerful effect on our physical life and our mood, just as hormones underlie male aggression and affect potency as men age. During the passage through menopause, when hormones are spiking and falling a few times every day, or possibly within an hour, many women do experience waves of fatigue and bouts of the blues. But that is very different from clinical depression. And most important, it is temporary.

In fact, women in their fifties, once through menopause, have the lowest rates of clinical depression compared with women at any other stage of life. Depression actually subsides with age for women.

Ironically, the people who are the most evasive and unsympathetic about menopause tend to be women in their forties; slouching towards the bridge to that unknown and frightening new territory of 'postmenopausal woman', they may be 'menophobic'. Their own resistance to identifying with the stage of life beyond reproductivity is sometimes expressed in an uncharacteristic intolerance of their own friends.

Menopause must be one of the most misunderstood passages in a woman's life. One study showed that two thirds of all American women say nothing to anybody as they approach what may be a distressing and even fearsome Change. But who can blame us? Menopause is inextricably linked with middle age. In the youth-oriented societies of North America and Europe, even the mention of middle age has a stigma about it. Shame, fear, and misinformation are the vague demons that have kept us silent about a passage that could not be more universal among females. The most common fears are: *I'll lose my looks, I'll lose my sex appeal, I'll get depressed, I'll become invisible*. We don't have to do any of these things. Yet the obvious sources of information and comfort – mothers, doctors, the media, academics – have shied away from the subject. All that is *beginning* to change. It is time to make this part of our public conversation, as natural a subject of discussion as pregnancy or male midlife crisis.

Right now, the number of American women in peri-menopause (the term used to designate the transition phase between regular periods and no periods at all), in menopause, or past menopause, totals *forty-three million*. The remainder of the decade will see an explosion in the menopausal population in the United States – the number of women between the ages of forty-five and fifty-four will increase by half, from 13 million to 19 million, by the year 2000. And over the next two decades, 40 to 50 million women will pass through the Change.

In Great Britain the 'age wave' is even farther along. At present, those fifty years old and over already represent one third of the total population of 55 million. A recent report for the Carnegie Inquiry into the Third Age counts the number of women currently over forty as 13 million, growing by another million and a half by the year 2001. The sheer numbers may at last confer normalcy on this predictable passage. But demographics aren't the only reason that our perceptions of the Change of Life are beginning to undergo radical alteration.

Menopause is no longer a marker that means This Way to The End. Today fifty is the apex of the female life cycle. And today, menopause is more properly seen as the gateway to a *second adulthood*, a series of stages never before part of the predictable life cycle for other than the very long-lived.

If forty-five is the old age of youth, fifty is the youth of a woman's second adulthood. In fact, we have the same number of years to look forward to as we have already lived as reproductive women. You don't believe it, do you? Consider. Most women begin menstruating at about thirteen and begin stopping at around forty-eight – remaining defined, and confined, to some degree by their procreative abilities for thirty-five years. The life expectancy of a woman fortunate enough to live to age fifty in the US or UK is now eighty-one. (A man of fifty can expect to live until seventy-six.) So, from the time she reaches perimenopause, the average woman has thirty-three more years. And an increasing number of women are living into advanced old age.

It is time to render normalcy to a normal physical process that ushers in the youth of our second adulthood. This is a passage as momentous as the one into adolescence. Indeed, the menopausal passage is almost the mirror image of the transition to adolescence for females, and it will take just as many years. Jolted into menstruating at twelve or thirteen – remember? – it took five years or more for our bodies to adjust to our uniquely altered chemistry, while our minds struggled to incorporate our new self-image. So, too, must we readjust to *not* menstruating.

Just as we were apprehensive as eleven-year-olds, standing on the doorstep of childhood, about to be pushed out into the unknown turbulence of puberty, so are we naturally nervous, at the approach of menopause, about letting go of aspects of femininity that have defined us. We become more acutely aware of health, appearance, economic security, and the harbingers of mortality.

I know what you're thinking. *Thank God this is a book that I don't have to read.* Because you're not fifty yet, or even close. That's the first misconception.

'YOU'RE NOT
OLD ENOUGH'

Murphy Brown may be having a baby in her forties, but Candice Bergen, who plays the successful anchorwoman on TV, is beginning to think about the Change of Life. The ravishing 46-year-old, having married late and blossomed both as a mother and a comedienne in her fifth decade, feels the shock of time compression. It came out in an interview with Jane Pauley on *Real Life*: 'I saw this article on menopause in a magazine and I went, well, I don't need to look at *that*,' and she wrinkled her Scandinavian ski-jump nose. 'And then I thought, "Oh, my *God*! Is this what's coming? Is this what's next? We have to deal with menopause? At my age? But I'm a *kid*."'

Menopause is arbitrarily defined as 'the final cessation of menstruation', as if it were a single point in time when the switch is turned off on those fabulous egg-ripening machines, the ovaries. In fact, it's a much more gradual, stop-start series of pauses in ovarian function that are part of that mysterious process called ageing. (A more comprehensive term is the climacteric, for which there is a male counterpart.) We are born with all the eggs we'll ever have, about seven hundred thousand. Each month after puberty, one ovary offers up a selection of from twenty to one thousand mature eggs, though usually only one is released into the fallopian tube to meet any sperm in the vicinity. As we get close to the bottom of the egg basket, ovulation doesn't always take place. The quality of egg follicles that month may be substandard, or there may not be sufficient oestrogen manufactured by the ovaries. When the supply of viable eggs is gone, menstruation stops completely and the fertile period of a woman's life ends.

The median age at which women in Western countries stop ovulating altogether is 50.8. But today there are no clear age cues to when the long transition begins, or when it ends. 'For a long time we've thought of menopause as a very sudden event – it really isn't,' says Dr Trudy Bush, epidemiologist and associate professor of obstetrics and gynaecology at Johns Hopkins Medical School. 'The ovaries start producing less oestrogen probably in the mid-thirties. There's a gradual loss of oestrogen production and other hormones until the ovaries finally stop putting out very much oestrogen at all. It's not uncommon to see symptoms in the early forties as a sign of gradual oestrogen withdrawal.'

Eight women out of every one hundred undergo a natural menopause *before age forty*, according to renowned reproductive endocrinologist Dr Lila Nachtigall, director of the Women's Wellness Division at New York School of Medicine. The youngest case on record was recently seen at Kings College Hospital: a nineteen-year-old girl.

Increasingly, say veteran practitioners, the American women turning up in menopause clinics are younger by four or five years than in the recent past. Researchers now admit they have underestimated the number of younger women who experience all the symptoms of menopause even though they still have periods. Some speculate that in the past, when women had many pregnancies, they had an easier menopause; as middle-class Western women have changed their life style – postponing childbirth, having fewer children, synthetically controlling their menstrual cycle and often introducing fertility drugs or having tubes tied or a uterus surgically removed – they may be throwing their hormonal systems out of balance. 'We know now there are women who start experiencing changes in their menstrual cycle in their late thirties,' says Phyllis Kernoff Mansfield, a veteran researcher of female cycles at Penn State.

My own younger sister started missing periods when she was forty-three – five years earlier than it began with me. One month her 'little friend' would come, then not again for another two or three months, whereupon it would reappear, only to disappear again. After half a year of this, feeling poorly, she called her gynaecologist and popped the obvious question: 'Is this the beginning of menopause?'

'No,' he stated categorically. 'You're not old enough.'

It's tempting to take this sop so commonly put out by physicians and to go away feeling smug and secure in one's continuing fecundity. Isn't it reassuring to know that you're still young? Well, not *young* exactly, but still, in some respect at least, *underage*.

'I started very early, at forty,' I was told by another woman I'll call Barbara, a delightfully wise Oregonian with a thriving psychotherapy practice. 'It was no fun. I was blown away by the hot flushes. I felt enormous restlessness, and cranky, cranky, cranky!' Her doctor, too, said she wasn't old enough to take oestrogen. Or, as she heard it, she hadn't suffered enough.

A roaring extrovert, Barbara stood up to her full five feet nine inches and stared down her doctor: 'Either you give me oestrogen, or the next time I have a hot flush I'm going to rip my clothes off and shout your name!'

The man dispensed the pills and preserved his anonymity, but once on hormones Barbara blew up. 'I gained five pounds a year for six years until I finally said the hell with it. I quit taking the oestrogen, and I have all the lines in my face to show for it.' Now in her early fifties, she does look parched and abruptly elderly. 'You age faster after menopause,' she concludes, though it would be more accurate to say that one ages faster after any *abrupt* withdrawal from hormones.

On the opposite end, women may never be quite sure when, or if, they have finished with menopause. This is particularly true for women who go right on to hormone therapy at the first signs of the Change and continue having periods as if they were still reproductive. There is no noticeable evidence of when they stop ovulating, no clear metaphysical marker that they are moving beyond fertility into another stage of life.

Margaret Mead originated the memorable phase *post-menopausal zest*. Yet Mary Catherine Bateson, the daughter of the pioneering anthropologist, is still puzzled about when her own mother actually became menopausal. When Dr Mead reached the age of forty-eight and probably experienced the first hot flushes, she persuaded her doctor to try giving her shots of oestrogen, the primary female hormone, telling him it was for a circulatory problem. 'And it worked,' she noted in a brief medical history made available to me by her daughter, an anthropological researcher and author in her own right. At age fifty-three Dr Mead noted 'longer space between periods and lower flow'. But she continued to have hormone-induced periods for another eight years, whereupon she asserted that she had held off menopause until her sixties.

To add to the age blurring, vanguard baby boomers are giving birth to yet another phenomenon unique to their generation: *menopause mums*. A woman I'll call Sondra describes herself as 'a classic Sixties person'. After graduating from Columbia University, she spent the next fifteen years as a politically obsessed radical in 'movement work', followed by a very respectable marriage and a cascade of miscarriages. Sondra was forty-two by the time she finally produced her first baby. That was two years ago.

'Thank God I finished breast feeding just in time for menopause,' she deadpanned. She swears she felt hot flushes while she was breast feeding (a normal occurrence).

Over the next few years the boardrooms of America are going to light up with hot flushes. The point women among the baby boomers, those now in their mid-forties who are the first among their generation to approach the passage into menopause, are probably operating at 110 percent. They may be in command positions in their professional life, or starting over to get a graduate degree, while also feeling a new sense of social obligation. Those who have remained childless and had conflicting feelings about it can turn their caregiving instincts outward. The married ones have a new chance for romance with a neglected husband, now that the nest is empty; the divorced or widowed ones may choose to savour their independence or delight in a new love, or a new sexual orientation. But at the same time, many women over forty-five are likely to be sandwiched between an abruptly dependent parent or in-law who is entering the twilight of ill health, and the continued dependence of children who today remain adolescent until the end of their twenties – and even move back in! This is no time suddenly to find one can't sleep, or can't shake the blues, or can't call up facts memorized the day before.

Moreover, acute or prolonged stress can affect a woman's cycle at any point in her life. Psychologist Ellen McGrath, a vivacious and experienced media spokeswoman in her midforties, was preparing to go out on her first book tour. She was petrified. She had drawn for three years on all her physical and mental resources to produce her magnum opus on depression, a book for the popular market titled *When Feeling Bad Is Good*. Now she had to go out and sell it; no tryouts out of town, she had to open on a national breakfast TV show before an audience of five million.

'The week before the tour, suddenly I couldn't remember my material. Pieces of it would just go. I thought, *My God, my mind is the main thing I have. What's happening to me?* Dr McGrath had recently been having trouble sleeping, feeling vaguely hot but without sweating. Earlier, I had shared with her some of my research. 'Though I never thought it would apply to me, I had some hunch of what this could be, and a name for my malaise – menopause.' So she asked her doctor to fit her in immediately and had a blood test done to measure her hormone levels. 'Turns out, I wasn't just in *peri*menopause. I had gone straight into full menopause, at forty-six!' The doctor gave her an injection of oestrogen to hold her over for several months. 'The astounding thing was, my symptoms disappeared within forty-eight hours,' says McGrath.

Unfortunately, women who begin the Change early may find their friends turn a cold shoulder; out of ignorance, perhaps, or because they feel threatened. 'I had the menopause in total isolation,' confesses Carmen Callil, the brilliant, bumptious managing director of the Chatto & Windus publishing label in London. Only ten when she entered menarche, she was forty-six when menopause 'descended like a cloud'.

Because she was so young, 'not a soul, not one of my friends, could talk to me about it.'

Walking home, the road would seem to her to move up and down. (Dizziness is not an uncommon symptom of fluctuating oestrogen levels.) Never known for her patience, Callil could not abide being made to wait in a shop. 'The irritability went over the top, followed by insomnia and depression.' Her doctor refused to believe that her symptoms indicated menopause. 'I must have gone six months to a year thinking I was going mad.'

One day, the editor was having a drink with writer Fay Weldon. 'You look rotten,' said the always-frank Weldon.

'I feel absolutely bloody awful,' Callil admitted, blurting out that it must be because of the menopause.

'You must go on hormones, immediately,' counselled Weldon.

That was seven years ago. Despite some unpleasant side effects, and cystic breasts which require her to have checkups every three months, Callil knows she would be a different person if it weren't for replacing her hormones.

'They can bury me with my little pills for the next world, like Tut,' she quips.

How long does she intend to live? I asked.

'Until about ninety,' she replies enthusiastically. 'My mother is eighty-seven, but her bones have gone, of course. It's a completely different generation.'

There is another reason that menopause is no longer clearly age-linked today. More than one third of the women in the United States have hysterectomies – thirty-seven women out of one hundred – an astounding figure. (North America leads the world in numbers of hysterectomies, with twice as many as in Great Britain.) The majority of these women have hysterectomies between the ages of twenty-five and forty-four. A classical hysterectomy, which means removal of the uterus and cervix, *even without removal of the ovaries,* usually brings on an early menopause, within two years of the surgery. Removal of the ovaries, called oophorectomy, brings on menopause immediately, no matter how young a woman is.

This is all part of a fundamental change in the way we view the adult life cycle of women. *The biological transition of menopause is no longer an age-tied marker event.*

But no matter when the first awareness dawns on a woman that menopause might be imminent for *her*, it comes as a shock. Virtually nothing prepares most women for this mysterious and momentous transition. Indeed, some of us unconsciously tell ourselves, 'It's not going to happen to me.'

WHEN YOU LEAST EXPECT IT

No more incongruous time or place could be imagined, the night I was hit by the first bombshell of the battle with menopause. It was a Sunday evening. Snug inside a remarriage not yet a year old, I was sitting utterly still, reading, in a velvet-covered armchair. A pillow's throw away my husband was doing the same, while jazz lapped at our ears and snow curtained the window. Every so often we looked up and congratulated ourselves on staying home in this cocoon of comfort and safeness and love we had created.

Then the little grenade went off in my brain. A flash, a shock, a sudden surge of electrical current that whizzed through my head and left me feeling shaken, nervous, off-balance.

'What was that?' I must have mumbled.

'What?'

'Nothing.'

But some powerful switch had been thrown. I tried to go back to reading. It was difficult to concentrate. When I looked down at the pages I had just finished, I realized the imprint of their content on my brain had washed out. I felt hot, then clammy. I tried lying down, but sleep could not soak up the agitation. My heart was racing, but from what? Complete repose? I felt, for perhaps the first time in my life since the age of thirteen, profoundly ill at ease inside my body.

In the months that followed, I sometimes felt *outside* of my body. I was aware of spates of 'static' in my brain, and came to recognize the aura which preceded the first migraine-like headaches I'd ever had. Usually optimistic, I began having little bouts of blues. Then little crashes of fatigue. Having always counted on abundant energy, it was profoundly upsetting to find myself sometimes crawling home from a day of writing and falling into bed for a 'nap', from which I had to drag myself up just to have dinner.

I was only forty-eight. And still menstruating. So this couldn't be 'Change of Life', could it?

Besides, all these strange physical sensations were only background noise in what was otherwise a thrilling, adrenalin-pumping, mind-stretching period of creative redirection, both in my career and my new family life. I was travelling all over the country and the world and coming home to a husband and new adopted child, both of whom I adored, satisfied that another beloved daughter was already launched. So I took Scarlett's 'fiddle-dee-dee' approach; I'd think about it to-morrow.

But tomorrow I began to notice something strange. For the first time since my early teens, when the sexual pilot light went on and I was warned not to want sex too much, I began to worry about not wanting it enough. Again, I had the sensation of standing outside my body and scolding it: 'What's the matter with you – why don't you *act* the way I feel any more?'

I went to see my conservative, male gynaecologist, known as a superb clinician but short on communication skills. He measured my hormone levels. I was very low on oestrogen. I vaguely remembered my family doctor having mentioned in passing, when he'd rattled off the results of my annual physical in recent years, that my oestrogen levels were getting lower and lower.

'Could I be a candidate for hormone replacement therapy?' I asked.

'Not yet.' My gynaecologist went strictly by the book. 'You're not in menopause because you're still menstruating. You have to be menstruation-free for a year before I can give you oestrogen replacement.'

'But this, um, effect on my sexual response' – embarrassed, I fumbled for the words – 'couldn't that be because I need more oestrogen, like a vitamin supplement?'

'It's nothing I can help you with. Decrease in sexual response is just a natural part of ageing.'

The curt clinician washed his hands of me. I left his office feeling as though I'd just been handed a one-way ticket to the dumpster. *Does this mean I can't be me any more?*

It was time for me to shop for another gynaecologist. A recommendation sent me to see Patricia Allen, a vivacious woman in her thirties and an attending physician at New York Hospital who demands excellence of herself and discipline from her patients. She made it clear from the start that she does not accept passive patients or women who smoke, only those who are willing to participate actively in their own health care. That sounded reasonable. She spent a good twenty minutes before the physical exam taking a holistic history. The irregular periods, the erratic expanding and constricting of blood vessels that caused the static, and the mood swings indicated to her that I was in perimenopause. Then she said something startling:

'I believe in treating each patient as an individual. This perimenopausal period should be a transformation, so that a woman gets to become – physically, emotionally, and spiritually – the best that she ever was.' Imagine your run-of-the-mill male gynaecologist harbouring such a radical point of view!

Dr Allen posited that the impact of low oestrogen on me, as on many women, was emotional. Of the several hundred patients who consult her about managing their menopause, quite a few mention feeling depressed although they have no rational reason to be. She also took seriously my distress over changes in libido. She asked if there was a history of osteoporosis in my family, which brought to mind memories of my mother suffering in her seventies as she sat on her powdery bones.

All in all, Dr Allen felt I was a good candidate for hormone therapy, but she drove a strict bargain with her patients. Oestrogen by itself carries a known increase in the risk of cancer of the endometrium – the lining of the uterus, which is sloughed during menstrual periods. So she also prescribed a synthetic progesterone as protection against that risk. Also, I would have to agree to have an endometrial biopsy several months later to detect any changes in the tissue. She also urged me to have a bone density evaluation done, as well as a mammogram. This complete diagnostic workup cost eight hundred dollars, much of which was reimbursable by health insurance. It was costly, but it turned out to be part of an investment in long-term health and productivity that has more than paid for itself – and one I would recommend for all women who can afford it.

But even this sympathetic gynaecologist, like every other clinician, was unable to give definitive answers concerning the increased risk of breast cancer when one takes hormones. 'We just don't know.'

I filled the standardized prescription for 0.625 mg of Premarin (oestrogen made from pregnant mares' urine, from which it derives its unforgettable name) and 10 mg tablets of Provera, a synthetic progesterone that stimulates the sloughing of the uterine lining. This is an approximation of the two hormones that the body produces naturally in the reproductive years.

After only a month, the oestrogen had rekindled sexual desire, stopped the surges of static and dips of fatigue, and chased away the blues. But the Provera was another matter. It brought on unbelievable physical and emotional symptoms that I'd never experienced before. After a year of the combined hormones, my body seemed to be at war with itself for half of every month. My energy was flagging, and resistance to minor infections was falling. I felt as if I were racing my motor. So I stopped taking hormones cold turkey.

Dr Allen agreed it was a good idea to take a break and see how the body responded. If nothing else, she said, going off hormones often serves to remind women why they started taking them in the first place.

For the first two months off hormones I felt marvellous; the bloating disappeared, as did the induced periods, and the terrible cramps and tensions and sleeplessness that had begun to accompany them. I even got my waist back. Then, a crash. All the perimenopausal phenomena returned with exaggerated force. Now the static became full-fledged hot flushes and night sweats that interrupted sleep and left me limp by morning. I went back to my oestrogen pills.

Within days the blue-meanie moods lifted. I was able to write for twelve hours straight on deadline, and remain calm and reasonable under crisis. Within a few weeks all the other complaints were gone. I was staggered by the potency of the female hormone.

But the impact of the progesterone was also intensified. On day fifteen, when I had to add the Provera pills to my regimen, I felt by afternoon as if I had a terrible hangover. This chemically induced state was not to be subdued by aspirin or a walk in the park. It only worsened as the day wore on, bringing with it a racing heart, irritability, waves of sadness, and difficulty concentrating. And to top it off, the hot flushes came back! Cramps introduced pain for a week at a time. By night, I couldn't go to sleep without a glass of wine, and even then was awakened by a racing heartbeat and sweating. *Won't I ever be me any more?*

It didn't require a ten-year clinical trial and double-blind study to guess what was going on. Taking synthetic progesterone for half of each month was like pushing down the gas pedal and putting on the brakes at the same time, and it had left my body confused and worn out.

Clinicians I later interviewed relayed common side effects reported by their patients who were taking the drug: 'Whenever I take that Provera I have migraines, bloating, breast tenderness, the blues, I feel awful and want to die.'

No wonder only 15 percent of American women in

menopause are getting hormone supplements. The numbers are even lower in Great Britain, where only 9 percent of women with menopausal symptoms are on hormone replacement therapy. Dr Marc Deitch, medical director of Wyeth-Ayerst, the cash cow of the pharmaceutical giant American Home Products, which introduced Premarin fifty years ago, acknowledges that the average length of time women continue on oestrogen replacement is only nine months. An estimated one third of those given prescriptions for hormones never even fill them, and two thirds of those who start out with the combination simply drop the synthetic progesterone after about a year.

My little truancy was to stop taking the nasty progesterone and keep on with my happy oestrogen pills. However, I cut the dose in half. Dr Allen warned me this was not conventional treatment, explaining again that in a woman with a uterus, if the supplemental oestrogen is not challenged with some form of progesterone, the risk of uterine cancer increases sixfold. It is now the consensus of the World College of Obstetricians and Gynecologists that if a proper progesterone is given with the oestrogen, there is no risk whatsoever of uterine cancer. It is also recognized that 0.3 mg of Premarin does not offer significant support to the bones.

'Why don't you do some research on other regimens,' Dr Allen suggested. Doctors who have done small-scale research report that synthetic progesterone blocks some of the oestrogen-receptor sites – so an internal war between the two hormones is an endocrinological reality! Synthetic progesterone therefore counters some of the cardio-protective effect that is one of the most highly touted benefits of oestrogen. A Swedish study, which showed oestrogen slightly increases a woman's risk of breast cancer, fingered the addition of progesterone drugs as possibly furthering the risk – and made a big splash in international newspapers. The study was bitterly criticized by North American experts for drawing conclusions from too small a sample of women who were given the oestrogen-progesterone combination.

Believe it or not, no published data existed in North America at the beginning of 1993 on the long-term carcinogenic effects on the breast of the combined hormone therapy routinely prescribed for women in menopause. I also found that Provera has never been approved for treatment of menopause by the US Food and Drug Administration. Notwithstanding, the FDA's Advisory Committee on Fertility and Maternal Health Drugs stated in 1991 that this combination of hormones 'may be used indefinitely by a woman with a uterus'. Asked what proportion of the female population over age fifty would be suitable candidates for long-term consumption of oestrogen alone or combined with synthetic progesterone, the committee replied 'Virtually all'. A blank cheque.

The latest information I have been able to uncover about progesterone is even more dismaying. The famous Swedish study by Berqvist and Persson originally exaggerated the increase in risk of breast cancer for women using hormone therapy. In a follow-up letter to *The Lancet* in late 1992, the researchers have corrected their numbers. What their data now shows is that the risk associated with long-term use of the *combination* of oestrogen and progesterone is higher than with oestrogen alone.

New biological laboratory evidence in the US also suggests that progesterone may increase the risk of breast cancer, according to a British bench scientist now at the University of Southern California, Malcolm Pike. He has demonstrated that while progesterone blocks the cancer-precursor effect of oestrogen in the uterus, it has the opposite effect on breast tissue. According to another of the experts at USC, cancer epidemiologist Dr Brian Henderson, 'if oestrogen increases the risk of breast cancer by 2 to 3 percent a year, adding up to about 25 percent over ten years – which is a reasonable summarization of the literature – then adding progesterone on a regular basis looks like it will double that risk. That would make it not a 25 percent but a 50 percent increase after ten years.'

In 1991, $750 million of oestrogen products were sold in the United States. Drug companies anticipate that these hormones will account for close to a billion-dollar market in 1992.

With the baby boom bulge projected to add over half a million women to the midlife population each year for the rest of the decade, the menopause market is becoming big business.

'The bottom line is the right studies need to be done for the right length of time, and, clearly, for economic and political reasons they're not,' says Dr Jamie Grifo, a gynaecologist at New York Hospital. 'Why? Who supports the majority of the research? The drug companies.'

Yet over the past few years hormone therapy has been routinely prescribed by doctors to somewhere between four and five million American women. Is it even conceivable that millions of men over fifty – those at the highest levels of the power structure – would be herded by physicians towards chemical dependence on powerful hormones at suspicion for causing testicular cancer? We are a generation of hormone guinea pigs. 'It's the largest *un*controlled clinical trial in the history of medicine,' charges public-health expert Dr Lewis Kuller. This was my introduction to the scandalous politics of menopause.

DEAL OR DENY?

My experience is not abnormal. From 10 to 15 percent of women are assumed by the few, inadequate studies to have no problems with menopause. Another 10 to 15 percent are rendered temporarily dysfunctional. The rest of us – 70 percent of all women – wrestle to some degree with difficulties that come and go over a period of years as we deal with the long transition from our reproductive state. (Data going back to the nineteenth century is consistent: almost all women experience some menopausal symptoms, but few have severe problems.)

The menopause experience varies with genes, age, class,

temperament, marital status, whether or not a woman has had children – everything. Antonia Fraser, the author of internationally acclaimed historical biographies, is a prime example of those fortunate women who are scarcely aware of the Change. When we met for lunch at the English Garden, I couldn't quite believe she had just turned sixty. A tall, strongly built woman who has borne six children and enjoyed a sexually robust past, Lady Antonia remains intensely feminine. From the gossamer blonde hair fluffed around her face and the flirtatious sweep of her opaline blue eyes, to the breathy voice that veils the perfectionism with which she chooses her words and crafts insights, she seems to sit very comfortably, and naturally, within her own skin. And enviable skin it is: 'lucky genes' keep it glistening like a freshly peeled pear. Fine tracings on either side of her lips and eyes are the only certain evidence of passing time. It isn't as though she has been resting on her laurels. She had spent the past two years working feverishly to finish her latest romantic historical biography, *The Six Wives of Henry VIII*, so that it could be published on her sixtieth birthday.

Some among the previous generation of women in her famous family had 'floods' during menopause. Lady Antonia had expected it would be the same for her. 'I didn't think it was worrying, it would just be extremely inconvenient.' As it transpired, her cycle stopped at the age of forty-nine. No signs. 'Nothing, except a slight tendency to throw open the windows for fresh air.'

Being the beaverish historian that she is, Lady Antonia had checked her recollection with her husband, Harold Pinter, the night before our interview. 'Am I fantasizing?' she asked. 'He might have said "You were bloody hell."'

But Harold had said, 'No, you're not fantasizing.'

She never considered taking hormones, feeling no need. But she keeps up regularly with her former flatmates from Oxford, and as they talked through menopause she learned there is a very wide range of experience. 'One of my closest friends had a very bad time with depression,' she recounts, 'and was saved by HRT. Her looks certainly improved on the hormones.' She smiles, self-deprecatingly, 'You know, you *can't* help looking and comparing.'

Even fortunates like the aristocratic Lady Antonia, however, do have the long-term health impact of the Change to consider.

'Menopause is not a disease,' says epidemiologist Trudy Bush. 'It's a life transition, but it carries with it a different internal hormonal milieu which is, in fact, detrimental to our bodies. When we don't have oestrogen our bones get brittle, our rates of heart disease go up, our vagina becomes less moist, our skin becomes dry and thin. In fact, we can reverse those processes that are related to the hormones rather than to ageing per se.'

Oestrogen is involved in something like three hundred bodily processes. So, when it dips below levels one's body has come to rely upon as normal for thirty years or more, the body is naturally thrown out of balance. The brain's brain, the hypothalamus, cannot coordinate with its usual precision functions like body temperature, metabolic rate, sleep cycle, blood chemistry, and so on.

Subtle influences on brain chemistry, similar to the experience of jet lag, may be a harbinger of perimenopause, for instance. The London editor, Eve Pollard, admits that she sometimes has a little more difficulty concentrating or remembering things these days. 'I know I have to make lists, but then I'm running a magazine and a newspaper and trying to manage children and step-children as they get older, when you can't lay down the law any more.' On her second marriage, juggling two children and three step-children, Ms Pollard may be in for a pleasant surprise. All but about 10 percent of women, which represents the extreme, will function quite effectively throughout menopause at balancing their usual nine lives. But they must take the trouble to inform themselves, since no one else will. 'All of us are quite ignorant,' Pollard admits.

The temptation, of course, is to deny the signs. Or to give up on dealing with the larger passage because we can't find quick and easy answers to resolve the physical challenge of menopause. In talking to women all over the country, I did find some significant differences in attitudes and reactions to menopause, depending on how women are valued in a particular subculture. But there was one strong common denominator: women in midlife are afraid to know – and fiercely resist acknowledging – that menopause can affect *them*; but at the same time, in spite of themselves, they are desperately anxious to learn what it's all about. Privately, they will go to extraordinary lengths to pick up information: cornering a researcher at a party and interrogating him, stealing books from doctors' offices (I was particularly proud to learn that *The Silent Passage* made the list of Ten Most Shoplifted Books in America) but heaven forbid that anyone should bring up the subject at the dinner table! Psychologist Abraham Maslow gave a name to this syndrome of ambivalence: 'the need to know and the fear of knowing'.

In fact, there is no single, risk-free solution that suits everyone. Menopause is highly idiosyncratic. Remember how different we were one from another as we entered puberty – some of us embarrassed still to be wearing vests at thirteen, while our best friend was turning into a hunchback to hide the pods suddenly swelling under her sweater? Well, the Change of Life is even more individual. Peggy Sue may tell you that she hardly noticed a thing. Her periods tapered off, she had a few hot flushes, but she sailed right through – no problem. Peggy Sue may be one of the lucky 10 or 15 percent of women who find the Change of Life uneventful. She may also be plump, or obese, and since oestrogen is stored in the fat cells this is one case where fat is more advantageous than thin.

Or, she may be lying.

Whatever Peggy Sue's experience of the Change, it doesn't make *your* signs and symptoms any less true. The older we grow, the more *un*like we are, one from another. Besides the changes in our brains and sexual characteristics over the years, our endocrine systems are different, our metabolism is different, our blood vessels and bones become more dissimilar, depending on our lifetime eating and exercise habits. So it is not surprising that there is not *one* menopause – there are hundreds of variations.

But instead of giving in to frustration over dealing with our uniqueness, we can recognize how lucky we are. In all of human history women's lives were under the coercion of their biology. Today we don't have to be forty-five years old and suddenly oestrogen deficient, miserable, and without recourse. We have choices. And they don't all involve taking drugs, by any means.

The first step we can take towards mastering this stage of life is to describe the beast, give a shape and characteristics to it, and look it in the face. The actual derivation of the word menopause is from the Greek *meno*, meaning 'month', and *pausis*, which is literally translated 'ending', though more accurately it connotes a pause in the life cycle. The Change of Life is one of the three great 'blood mysteries' that demarcate a woman's inner life, the earlier ones being menarche and pregnancy. Despite the trial-and-error state of medical care, a woman at fifty now has a second chance. To use it, she must make an alliance with her body and negotiate with her vanity. Today's healthy, active pace-setters will become the pioneers, mapping out a whole new territory for potent living and wisdom-sharing from one's fifties to one's eighties and even beyond.

Yet the reluctance to discuss both the trials and rewards of moving through the Change of Life has obscured the facts, often keeping younger women in a state of menopausal dread. One naturally asks, *If menopause is such a significant passage to a whole new stage of life, why is it so neglected?*

MOTHER DOESN'T
KNOW BEST

⤜⤚

'I don't know how to be fifty,' one West Coast woman told me. 'I'm not going to be fifty like my mother, and there haven't really been any models.'

Very rarely had any of the women I interviewed learned much about menopause from their own mothers. If they reported any mother-daughter conversation on the subject at all, the mothers' answers tended to be brief and evasive: 'There was nothing to it; my periods just stopped'; or 'I don't remember much about menopause'.

Not surprising. It was common in their day for women in the Change to be institutionalized. 'Nervous breakdown' they called it. Because nobody associated their intense depression with menopause and the *temporary* breakdown of hormonal balance.

In a longitudinal study of five hundred women graduates of a midwestern university, Professor Phyllis Mansfield found that college-educated women get their 'facts' about menopause first from a friend, second from books or the media, and only third from their mothers. The last person most women consult is a doctor. One woman told a researcher she learned about menopause from Edith on an episode of *All in the Family*.

There are good reasons that the same mothers and mothers-in-law who assume possession of the revealed wisdom on child rearing are peculiarly scanty of expertise on this subject. The mothers of today's menopause-aged women were an exceptionally prudish lot. It was shameful to discuss any bodily functions in their day.

And what was there to discuss about menopause? Our

mothers had no information. No biomedical research had been done into the most pressing health questions of women as they age. Most of our mothers had no idea of the major killer diseases or disorders that would deprive them of a decent quality of life in their sixties, seventies or eighties. And they certainly didn't know that their risk of being attacked by heart disease, hip fractures, and breast cancer was decidedly affected by the way they handled their Change of Life.

It is safe to assume most of our mothers never even heard the word 'osteoporosis' – a silent disease caused by deterioration of the bone tissue – much less associated it with menopause. Only in the last five years or so has osteoporosis been identified as a crippler of life's quality, afflicting almost twenty-five million women. It leeches the very lining of our bones, like a colony of termites inside our foundations. Beginning their invisible destruction as soon as our supply of oestrogen is depleted, these 'termites' accelerate their robbing of mineral from our bones during the time around menopause.

Many women in their forties today are at the hub of several generations. Unless they're incapacitated, they feel too stretched for time and money to consult doctors or take expensive tests in order to manage their own menopause. In fact, most middle-class and low-income women don't consult any professional about how to protect their health and wellbeing during the Change of Life. If they adopt their mothers' attitudes without examination, they often follow blindly a path that, unbeknownst to the older women, may have been responsible for untold deficits of mental and physical wellbeing.

In addition to the lack of informed guidance by their mothers, many women who are in the menopause years right now are handicapped by their own inhibitions. Born in the late thirties or early forties, they went through secondary in the uptight fifties, before the sexual revolution, before liberation, when only 'bad girls' became sexually active before marriage, and a lot of others lied about it. Part of what Americans call the Silent Generation, they have never been comfortable talking about sexual matters. Their silence on the subject of menopause may be an anachronism.

EVOLUTION AND THE VICTORIAN HANGOVER

Another reason for the mystery surrounding menopause is that human females today are monkeying with evolution. Most higher primates do not live long enough in the wild even to have a menopause; the phenomenon has never been clearly established in apes or monkeys, according to Kim Wallen, a researcher at Emory University's Yerkes Primate Center. Most female animals just go right on breeding until they roll over and die.

The same was true of human females for many thousands of years. At the turn of the century, an American woman could expect to live to the age of forty-seven or -eight. She bore an average of eight children, which kept her busy giving birth or nursing right up to menopause.

Nature, then, never provided for women who would *routinely* live several decades beyond the age of fifty. Once females had made their genetic contribution, evolution was finished with them, and society followed suit. Given this historically powerful linkage of menopause with decline and death, is it any wonder that today's women approach fifty under a shadow of archetypal fears of being transformed, all at once, into Old Woman?

The secrecy, shame and ignorance that still veil this natural transition have carried over from the Victorian age with very little mitigation of the punishing stereotypes. 'Menopause in the nineteenth century was described only in terms of what women lose at this stage of life,' says Marilyn Yalom, senior scholar at the Stanford University Institute for Research on Women and Gender. The Victorians were obsessed with women as reproductive creatures. Once barren and widowed, as they were likely to be by fifty, they were cued to view menopause as 'the gateway to old age through which a woman passed at the peril of her life'. Yalom's chapter in the documentary text, *Victorian Women*, quotes nineteenth-century obstetricians who taught that 'the Change of Life unhinges the female nervous system and deprives women of their personal charm'.

These attitudes were tempered somewhat by the sassy and energetic social activists who emerged between 1890 and 1920, a period that celebrated 'the renaissance of the middle-aged'. As death in childbirth was reduced, middle-class women began to appreciate the possibilities of a full life cycle and to cluster their childbearing in the earlier years of marriage. In their mature years they took up social causes, marched in parades, and founded movements. The great feminist leaders such as Elizabeth Cady Stanton celebrated the liberation of being in their fifties and continued as activists well into their sixties. *Cosmopolitan* magazine sang the praises of vital women of menopausal age in 1903: 'The woman of fifty who only a few years ago would have been sent to the ranks of dowagers and grandmothers, today is celebrated for distinctive charm and beauty, ripe views, disciplined intellect, cultivated and manifold gifts.' Once the twenties got underway, however, the former stereotypes resurfaced.

The most famed and prolific women writers over the past hundred years have largely ignored, or been ignorant of, menopause. The romantic novels of George Sand, one of the most staggeringly prolific writers of the nineteenth century in the French language, were read as widely as Balzac's and Hugo's throughout the European continent. Sand also penned twenty-five volumes of letters while inspiring the music of her younger lover, Frédéric Chopin. Yet in this vast landscape of words scholar Marilyn Yalom has uncovered only two personal letters in which Sand refers to the symptoms of menopause. In the first, written to her editor, Hetzel, in 1853, Sand was forty-nine years old:

> I am as well as I can be, given the crisis of my age. So far everything has taken place without grave consequence, but with sweats that I find overwhelming, and which are laughable because they are imaginary. I experience the phenomenon of believing that I am sweating 15 or 20 times a day and night ... I have both the heat and the fatigue. I wipe my face with a white handkerchief and it is laughable because I am not sweating at all. However, that makes me very tired.

Sand was chiding herself out of ignorance for having hot flushes and night sweats. Often, a woman does not perspire, even though she is experiencing an abrupt leap in skin temperature of one or two degrees. 'Even today, it's very difficult to explain to a woman that it's a real neuro-physiological event, not a psychological event at all, and therefore nothing she should be ashamed of,' says Dr Robert Lindsay, an endocrinologist and leading researcher in the field of menopausal medicine at the Helen Hayes Bone Center in West Haverstraw, New York. Not until the mid-1970s were laboratory tests developed that could demonstrate objectively the neurological discharge in the brain that causes the subjective changes women describe. When a woman says, 'I am now having a hot flush,' a machine similar to an EKG will show a spike in the ink line running across it.

George Sand refused to allow this inconvenience to interrupt her productivity and finished her letter by saying, 'Nonetheless I am working and I've just done a play in three acts ...' Weeks later she indicated in a letter to her son that she had 'rounded the horn' and felt better than she had for a long time. Sand was smart enough to know that even she should make a healthy adaptation in the exhausting nocturnal work habits she had devised, as a young mother, to work around domestic duties.

> I sleep well, I eat well, I no longer have those flushes and I'm working without fatigue. It is true that I don't

give myself to excess anymore and at one o' clock in the
morning I wrap myself in my bed without hesitation.

One in the morning, for George Sand, was early. After fifty,
she stopped writing from midnight to 4 a.m. But by then she
was a polished professional with twenty years of writing
behind her, and she was able to ensconce herself at her country
estate and produce the many novels for which she is famous.
George Sand was still vibrant, and still writing, when she died
at the age of seventy-two.

Anaïs Nin, another fearless watchwoman over the back
alleys of the female psyche, neglected the subject in her
writings. Virginia Woolf's fragile nature was bedevilled by
physical illness and mental anguish at every stage. She
attracted particularly harsh criticism for the book that
expressed her viewpoint as a woman in her fifties, *Three
Guineas*. Woolf attributed none of her ills to menopause, and
never mentioned it in her writings, though she must have
passed through it before she took her own life at fifty-nine.
Colette was one of the rare writers to mention menopause at
all in her work, portraying it in her novel *Break of Day* as both
daunting and potentially empowering.

The contemporary novelist, Barbara Taylor Bradford, who
writes hugely popular sagas about women who overcome
obstacles of class and culture, was startled when I asked her
if any of her heroines had ever had menopause.

'Why, no, I haven't given them menopause,' she said, adding 'that's interesting, now that you mention it, since Emma
[the inspiring heroine of *A Woman of Substance*] was in her
eighties.'

My hunch was that, like many earlier writers, she hadn't let
her characters have menopause because she didn't intend to
have it herself. Bradford had had an early menarche and was
determined not to pay any attention to the menopause when
it came round.

'I don't have time to dwell on things like that,' she told
herself, driving herself even harder when it did happen. She
is married and has no children. 'I was about forty-five or six.

The only sign I had was hot flushes. They started suddenly, out of the blue, and lasted three and a half years. As I think back, there was a sense of panic. I guess it was the menopause?'

A woman who feels too threatened to deal with the Change may experience a period of free-fall, accompanied by the kind of panic Bradford recalls. Her symptoms, minor though they were, challenged her belief that she would be immune to age-ing. Her way of coping was to shut herself in her writing room for twelve hours a day. She never wondered about her mother's death from heart failure or about protecting her bones. But after our conversation, she read up on the subject and called me a week later. She had decided to talk to her doctor about going on hormones. 'If I take them, it would be for long-term health reasons – heart and bone.'

With the Change now some seven years behind her, Barbara Taylor Bradford rivals the indefatigability of George Sand. She writes more, exercises more, and enjoys life more. 'I have more energy than when I was in my twenties!' she marvels. 'This is such a period of fruitfulness and fulfilment in a woman's life. I want people to know they shouldn't be afraid.'

Sounds like another woman who has 'rounded the horn' and found the euphoria that makes the trip worthwhile.

WOMEN ENTERING
THE ENLIGHTENED AGE

Is biology destiny? Of course not. But there are militant defenders of the opposing doctrine of 'cultural determinism' who want us to believe that, beneath the learned male and female roles that culture lays upon us, all people are essentially similar. Understandably, there is strong resistance to believing that our behaviour is influenced by the biochemical balance in our bodies, because it suggests that we have very little free will. It's unfortunate, and silly, to make it an either/or argument. If you ask me, do I believe in free will? I would borrow the answer given by Isaac Bashevis Singer. 'Of course, I have no choice.'

To writers like Barbara Ehrenreich, however, any honest examination of the hormonal differences between women and men – or between women and other women, for that matter – is dismissed as a surrender to the old biology-as-destiny credo. The cessation of menses, she wants us to believe, is 'an obvious nonevent'. (Like puberty, I suppose.) Menopause isn't an event at all, but a *process* that takes place over five to seven years and has as many profound metaphysical, social, and sexual layers of meaning as the passage of menarche, which ushers in a woman's fertility.

These polemicists seriously misrepresent the fledgling movement to bring menopause out of the closet. Beware of this logic when you encounter it. The proponents are often women frozen in an outdated era of feminism. Ignoring a host of new data that demonstrate some clear gender differences stemming, at least in part, from variations in male/female biology, they represent their views as a higher good than the truth. It can make them more dangerous than the wrong drug.

Animal studies have shown how fickle behaviour can be, depending upon the amount of male or female hormone present in either sex. Strong evidence already exists connecting the aggressive behaviour of males with the male hormone, testosterone. The more startling observations come from very recent studies of hyenas at the University of California, Berkeley. With other animals, male babies engage in more rough play than females, due to the early testosterone they had circulating during fetal life. In a unique situation in all of biology, the hormonal bath in which female hyena fetuses grow is loaded with oestrogen *and* testosterone, as well as androsteindione, a precursor able to be transformed into more fiery doses of testosterone. The females develop a huge clitoris at birth and eventually display a hanging genital that has erections and is indistinguishable from a male penis.

At the hyena pen in Berkeley, I watched the amazing gender-bending behaviour that results from this biological switch. No sooner were they born, than two females began tearing each other apart. When the third female of triplets emerged, she was barely an hour old before her sisters began chewing at her birth sack. The point was observable before our very eyes: high testosterone accounts for aggressive behaviour in both males and females.

As they age, the female hyenas' level of testosterone dips well below that of the males'. Notwithstanding, the females continue to be the more pugnacious and to remain in charge of their animal hierarchy. Dr Lawrence Frank and Dr Steven Glickman, animal behaviourists coordinating the study, tossed a huge hunk of horse meat into the pen of the young adults. The ranking female leapt on it and began reducing it to a grease spot, while the male lay back, passively, until she'd had her fill. 'At this point, he defers to her without giving it a second thought,' observed Dr Glickman. By then, learned behaviour has taken over from hormones. Thus does it remain difficult to disentangle culture from hormonal effects.

A clear link has been established, for example, between oestrogen and women's verbal superiority, just as there is a link between testosterone and men's facility with maths and visual-spatial tasks. The levels of hormone matter as well. When women of reproductive age were studied recently, their verbal – and manual – dexterity was found to peak in the middle of their monthly cycle – just when oestrogen levels were at their highest. Immediately after they finished menstruating, when circulating oestrogen was at its lowest monthly ebb, their speed on verbal tasks declined. Even at their lowest speed, however, most of the women outperformed men on all verbal tests. By the same token, pubescent boys who have abnormally low levels of testosterone do poorly on spatial tasks.

In pulling together these recent studies, anthropologist Helen E. Fisher, author of *Anatomy of Love: The Natural History of Monogamy, Adultery, and Divorce*, proposes that these subtle gender differences make evolutionary sense. When ancestral males squatted in the African veldt to watch and hunt animals many millennia ago, those who were best in the visual-spatial skills of mapping and tracking might well have survived disproportionately. Similarly, ancestral women needed minute manual dexterity to pick seeds and berries out of the dense vegetation, while verbal skills may have been critical to communicating with their young, again, selecting for these traits in modern women.

'For decades, if not centuries, scientists in search of an understanding of human nature have used male behaviour as a bench mark and compared all data on females with this standard,' writes Fisher, pointing out that this is why we have known almost nothing about the biological tendencies of women. Now that we are just beginning to learn, it would be a shame to throw out the baby with the ancestral bathwater. Fisher makes a good case from anthropological findings that the two sexes survived by teaming up and sharing one another's biological advantages. '. . . our ancestors had begun to collect, butcher, and share meat. The sexes had started to make their living as a team . . . this hunting-gathering life style would produce an intricate balance between women, men and power.'

The question inevitably comes up, is there a male menopause? Not precisely. All men do not become infertile at around the same age, and some men continue to have sufficient testosterone to sire children well into older age. Nevertheless, according to leading endocrinologists I have consulted, a decline in sexual prowess is a clear phenomenon among men, and it is correlated with a decline in testosterone levels. Dr Pentti Siiteri, former professor and co-director of the Reproductive Endocrinology Center at the University of California at San Francisco, and an authority on hormonal mechanisms, explains, 'This is analogous to what happens to a female, the significant difference being there is no sharp demarcation point; therefore, it is impossible to define when the decline in sexual prowess starts. Most men,' he adds, 'begin to taper off in their mid-fifties to sixties.'

But they don't talk about it. Not to their wives. Not even to other men. 'Because you don't want to admit weakening,' adds Dr Frank, 'your job as a male is to be strong.'

'Sooner or later, however, virtually all men will have a male menopause,' states Dr Siiteri. 'It's the difference between a gradual decline and a more abrupt one.'

Now here's the good news for women. Biology at the Change of Life works to women's advantage. The turmoil wrought by menopause mixes up the hormonal cocktail in new and different proportions. As the levels of the primary female hormone, oestrogen, continually decline, the chaser of male hormone, testosterone, increases in ratio. Before menopause, the average woman's level of testosterone is roughly 300 picograms. After a woman goes through the Change, if her ovaries are still intact, her testosterone level falls from 300 to about 215–220 – or one third. (If her ovaries are removed, the drop is to about 100, or a two-thirds fall.) At the same time, her oestrogen levels fall twelve-fold, a far greater decrease than that in the male hormone. And after the Change, her oestrogen levels remain fairly constant.

'Therefore, a postmenopausal woman has twenty times as much testosterone as a premenopausal woman,' concludes Dr Howard Judd, professor of Ob-Gyn at University of California, Los Angeles, whose scientific studies established these norms in the early 1970s.

This provides a biological basis that would explain, at least in part, the widespread phenomenon of post-menopausal zest and the greater assertiveness recorded, cross-culturally, among postmenopausal women. Aggressiveness is rooted in the male hormone testosterone and found in elevated levels in men and male baboons of high rank.

Hence, in many societies, middle-aged women – freed from the role of breeder and fired up with relatively higher levels of testosterone – rise in rank and power, in political, religious, economic and community life. Margaret Mead, a mentor of mine, summed it up in one sentence: 'There is no greater power in the world than the zest of a post-menopausal woman.'

Indeed, the most powerful woman in the world throughout the decade of the eighties was a menopausal woman. Margaret Thatcher was just about fifty when she broke the glass ceiling in Brit:sh politics and became leader of the Conservative Party. She went through menopause while making the leap to world leader. Eleanor Roosevelt, Golda Meir, and Indira Gandhi all came into their own in their postmenopausal years.

Today, many more women are rising to high levels in public life in Europe and America, and without having to be honorary males. Among the hundred women in the European Parliament are some very glamorous ladies indeed. The British House of Commons now seats sixty women. The first woman to sit on the US Supreme Court, Sandra Day O'Connor, and the first woman governor of Texas, the salty-tongued Anne Richards, are prime examples of strong-minded women with plenty of postmenopausal zest. Nine of the eleven women nominated by their parties to run for US Senate seats in the '92 election were in their fifties. Across Europe and North America there seems to be a new recognition: you don't have to be old and grey and male to be knowledgeable. You can be fifty and female and fabulous.

The sense of empowerment is not limited to upper-middle-class women or those in public life. The proportion of women in the British work force has risen during the long recession to 48 percent. Close to one quarter of the women earners in their fifties also act as unpaid health carers for elderly relatives or a sick husband. 'We were astonished to find that such a high proportion of them had full-time jobs,' confesses British MP Edwina Currie. 'When you asked them why, they said, "Well, I had to retain my sanity somehow."'

These are likely to be women who seek out hormone replacement and who, with their renewed vitality and self-confidence, burst out of old constraints. 'It's all part of having more money in their pockets, the kids having gone, the mortgage being close to paid off,' as Currie describes the new prototype of her middle-aged female constituents. 'They've gone for better promotions, they're working full time, and they know the boss needs them. Ten years ago they would sit quietly during a political meeting and look at their nails. Now they ask the fiercest questions I get. It's a total sea change of attitude amongst women of our age group.'

It would be remiss of me to represent all contemporary women in their middle years as similarly enlightened. Indeed, some of those with readiest access to the facts of life about the postmenopausal years are the most confused by the politicized debate over HRT. Some bury their heads in the sand and refuse to know what they know, or do much about it.

DOCTORS STILL IN
THE DARK AGES

Lamentably, few doctors are well-informed about menopause, and many assume the vaguely described symptoms are psychological in nature. Since physicians are temperamentally disposed to helping people, they, too, feel frustration over the state of scientific ignorance about women's health in the middle years.

'You don't need to know about that yet,' is one standard answer women are given. The doctor pats her on the head and out the door she goes, with her migrainous headaches, ill-defined blues, or unexplained fatigue – what could it be?

When one goes to a GP in Britain with vague menopausal complaints, one is in the lap of the gods. 'The vast majority of our GPs have not really known what to do about menopausal symptoms or HRT or osteoporosis, so what they've been doing is not much,' observes Linda Edwards, deputy director of the National Osteoporosis Society. Where health care is free, preventive medicine is not encouraged because it would be too costly.

'Our health service is very basic,' says Jean Shapiro, editor of *Ourselves Growing Older*. 'With government cuts and a reorganization of the health service into a business, doctors have less than ten minutes to see a patient. So you present one particular symptom, and you are lucky if even that is dealt with; quite a lot is missed, or dismissed as insignificant.'

Women who say, 'I feel down,' or 'I've got these awful headaches,' will most likely be given antidepressants, says Shapiro. It's a good way of getting rid of the patient. Except that antidepressants have no effect on menopause.

So often American women say, 'I'm waiting for my doctor to tell me what to do.' More commonly, she won't even bring up menopause, and her gynaecologist won't either. Some women spend the next three or five years making the rounds of internists, neurologists, even psychiatrists, with no resolution, because they all ignore the obvious.

The experience of a busy professional political activist in Washington is emblematic. Noticing her periods were scanty and intermittent and feeling uncharacteristically draggy, she went to her internist and plunked down $300 for a complete physical. She was forty-nine. The physician took a considerable amount of blood for tests. The results shed no light on her condition. Only when the activist talked to a woman friend who asked, 'What about your oestrogen level?' did the lightbulb flash on. She realized her doctor had not taken any hormone levels. He had never even mentioned menopause.

'The most important change going on in the body of a 49-year-old woman was never addressed,' she says, chagrined at her own passivity. 'Doctors treat our bodies as though we're the same machines as men, and we're not.'

'It wouldn't occur to a British woman to go to a gynaecologist unless there was something really wrong,' Fay Weldon told me. 'Besides, you don't want men looking up you.'

While it rings to my American ears quaintly Victorian to avoid 'men looking up you' (wouldn't that make delivering babies inconvenient?), I quite agree with Weldon that male doctors aren't likely to know more about a woman's body than she does. Nearly half the graduates coming out of British medical schools today are women, and they tend to be more sympathetic. Notwithstanding, a woman's own signs are her best guide as to whether or not she is nearing menopause or what phase of the long transition she might be in, and whether it is causing her problems. But in order to recognize those signs, and deal with each appropriately, *we must be educated*. It will not do to retreat behind the defence, *If I don't acknowledge it, it doesn't exist.*

Private gynaecologists by and large find the menopausal woman an unappealing patient. She isn't going to have any more babies. Apart from a hysterectomy, there is little chance she will require surgery – the moneymaking part of the practice – but she can be expected to complain about vague symptoms and ask questions for which even the sympathetic physician has only unsatisfactory answers. With candour, a dedicated female gynaecologist describes the attitudes of many of her male colleagues. 'They find us tedious because we're going to take up their time, and threatening because we're smart and we're grownups, we don't want any of their bullshit.'

Some doctors, like John Studd, a Harley Street practitioner, have made a brisk business out of menopause medicine. Dr Studd introduced the debate on HRT in the UK. He has earned a controversial reputation by recommending to his menopausal patients that they accept testosterone implants, along with oestrogen. Some of his former patients complain of an overstimulated sexual appetite; according to Germaine Greer it gave her an understanding of how a rapist feels.

A racing journalist from Suffolk described her experience. She had been feeling dozy, looking dehydrated, and was having difficulty concentrating; well, those could just be age, she told herself. 'But the real sign that scared me was a sort of drying up of the vagina,' she told me. Her male GP had brushed off her symptoms: there was nothing to be done for menopause. So she went off to see a private gynaecologist, who tested her hormone levels and did an examination.

'Atrophy!' he barked at her in his bombastic voice.

She did not think this diagnosis charming.

'Implant,' ordered the doctor.

The journalist backed off; she wasn't about to have a drug she couldn't control take up residence in her body for three months. So back she went to her GP to ask for the standard hormone calendar pack doled out by the Health Service, Prempak-C. It's administered like a one-size-fits-all item (although it does come in two strengths). The big pills, which are Premarin, made her feel better. But the little pills added for the last ten or twelve days (a synthetic progesterone called Norgestrel) made her breasts sore and produced almost continuous bleeding. Sick of the nuisance, she dropped the whole thing.

It's a typical story, says the osteoporosis expert, Linda Edwards. Women are often given HRT with only minimal advice. Not expecting side effects, they get nervous. Most GPs don't know how, or make no attempt, to tailor the type of hormone and regimen to the particular woman's chemistry. So when she complains, the GP simply shrugs and says, 'Well, obviously HRT doesn't suit you.'

The point is that there are almost a dozen different hormone preparations available in Europe; they can be delivered in varied combinations by pill, patch, injection, implant, cream, and with a regimen that does *not* produce withdrawal bleeding. (See chapter *Should I Or Shouldn't I?*) But a woman must not expect to go to a GP and get a magic bullet that will restore her body's balance like *that*. She should expect *at least a year* of trial and error before she finds the most comfortable routine to relieve her particular symptoms and protect her bones, heart, sexual energy and comfort, and her mental wellbeing.

The busy doctor of either sex in any country is likely to take an incomplete family history of the factors that impinge on menopause. Just how cursory these conversations can be is illustrated by the experience of a well-known columnist and her sister, both hard on age fifty. They consulted the same gynaecologist in the Boston area to ask what to do. Despite their genetic likeness, one was told she was a good candidate for hormones. Her sister was cautioned not to take hormones. It turns out that the sisters had emphasized different subjective fears. Senior American congresswoman Patricia Schroeder of Colorado, active in the campaign for women's health research and funding, cracks that 'If you get six menopausal women together, you'll find that their doctors are doing six different things. Our joke is that you might as well go to a veterinarian.'

There is a simple blood test a woman can ask for that is quite reliable in determining whether or not, and at what stage, she is in menopause. One should ask to have one's LH and FSH measured, along with the level of oestrogen. FSH, a follicle-stimulating hormone, and LH, a luteinizing hormone, are responsible for ovulation and under the control of the hormones oestrogen and progesterone. If the FSH and LH are both high, in the presence of low oestrogen, it is indicative of menopause.

THE HYSTERECTOMY TRAP

Hysterectomies are the second most common surgery for women in America, where the proliferation of this surgery is more than double the rate in most European countries. It is not even known exactly how many hysterectomies are performed on women each year in the US, because there is no organization that keeps national statistics on hysterectomies. In fact, the National Center for Health Statistics does not have a department that deals specifically with gynaecological issues. But the generally accepted estimate is that one out of three American women will surrender her womb to the surgeon's knife – usually between the ages of twenty-five and forty-four.

A mere 11 percent of the menopause surgeries performed in the US are done in response to a cancerous growth. Notwithstanding, there is growing pressure from some gynaecologists who urge women to consider a 'prophylactic hysterectomy'; that is, to undergo major surgery *on the chance* that at some future time she might develop cancer in her reproductive organs. A stylish ob-gyn man in Beverly Hills recommends prophylactic hysterectomies along with removal of the ovaries when his patients reach menopause.

A Seattle divorcee brags about solving the whole dilemma by having just such an elective hysterectomy at the age of forty-one. 'My doctor was a yanker instead of a saver,' she quips. 'But I wasn't going to use the equipment any more, I didn't want it. I'm glad I got rid of my ovaries.'

It may sound like a nice midlife housecleaning, but that brings us to another myth about the Change: if you have a hysterectomy, you bypass menopause. In fact, the latest research in Great Britain suggests just the opposite. 'If a woman has a hysterectomy, *even if her ovaries are conserved*, she will have a menopause within a couple of years,' according to Linda Edwards, deputy director of the National Osteoporosis Society in Bath.

A case in point is the story of a Rochester woman I interviewed, a college professor in the social sciences. Virginia, who requested anonymity, was seen by her family and friends and colleagues as a super-coper. At the age of forty-seven, she separated from her husband. She went into perimenopause at the same time, but she didn't know it.

'I was agitated all the time,' she recalls, looking back. 'I thought I was losing my memory. I had night sweats and blurred vision. Sometimes I'd be so fatigued, coming home from school, my legs would fold underneath me climbing up the stairs.'

And then came the all-too-common admission: 'I thought, because I'd had a hysterectomy, I wouldn't *have* a menopause.' Virginia never asked her doctor. And her doctor, a woman GP, said nothing to enlighten her. So, how did she manage?

Virginia would get into her car after work, two or three

times a week, and drive an hour and a half to Buffalo. There, unrecognized, invisible, she could sit in a shopping mall, and cry.

'I was like two people,' she recalls with anguish. Back home again, she would get stroked for being a super-coper. Only recently, in Virginia's fifty-second year, her doctor finally did blood tests to measure her hormone levels, and announced: 'Virginia, you're finished with menopause.'

It was the first time the subject had come up.

If both a woman's ovaries are removed, she will go into instant menopause. It is actually castration. Twice as many women who have a hysterectomy today, compared with twenty years ago, also have their ovaries removed. For a woman with a persistent ovarian tumour, it is common and necessary to have at least one ovary removed. However, before having both ovaries removed, a woman should be warned that the abrupt and total, rather than gradual, shutting down of ovarian function can be devastating, placing her at risk of serious depression. It also extinguishes sexual desire. Unless a woman immediately starts hormone replacement therapy and commits to remaining on the medication indefinitely, she will have all the symptoms of menopause, whatever her age. What's more, early surgical removal of the ovaries *doubles* the risk of osteoporosis. If you lose your ovaries at age thirty, by the time you reach age fifty your *bone age* may be seventy. Yet doctors often refuse to warn a woman that the surgery can have such lifelong effects even after the body heals.

I ran into this same high-handed attitude in a heavily utilized menopause clinic in the heart of London. When women complain about side effects from progesterone drugs, this doctor, like many, will often recommend a hysterectomy. He explains that it will free them from having to take the progesterone to protect their uterus. I asked if he would routinely take the ovaries as well?

'In a postmenopausal woman, the ovaries are of no use anyway,' he replied dismissively. I expressed alarm. Wasn't this extreme? The doctor was ignoring the fact that the ovaries continue to produce testosterone, which strongly influences a woman's sexual desire and energy.

'To a lot of people that seems like using a sledgehammer to open a nut,' he granted. 'But for patients who suffer badly, and desperately want to continue their HRT – especially women in their early to middle forties who are faced with this for another ten years – they say, "God, I can't take these side effects any more, take it all away."' He boasted that all such women, convinced by him to go ahead with a hysterectomy, 'thought it was the best thing since sliced bread.'

How much did he question women about their sexual pleasure and comfort, a year after performing these hysterectomies? I inquired.

'I must admit, personally speaking, not a great deal,' the surgeon said. 'Mrs Smith comes in, has a hysterectomy, you see her six or eight weeks later, and if she's making a satisfactory recovery, you don't see her again.'

'The concept that the ovary burns out is not true,' claims one of the experts on the postmenopausal ovary, Dr Howard Judd at UCLA. Although a woman's ovaries stop producing oestrogen, in postmenopause, they continue to produce a significant amount of testosterone.

A study that did take the trouble to reconsider the impact on sex life following a hysterectomy found that between 33 and 46 percent of the women whose ovaries had also been removed complained of reduced sexual responsiveness.

Fibroids often lead women to unnecessary hysterectomies. These benign growths are found in 20 percent of all women. (Fibroids are far more common among black women than white women, according to the National Black Women's Health Project.) Although the popularity of hysterectomy is highest in the South – 'Mississippi Appendectomy' it's called – and lowest in the Northeast where statistically there are more educated women, it is very common for women to mistake the normal symptoms of perimenopause for a more serious problem. Here is a typical scenario from the Massachusetts Women's Health Study of twenty-five thousand women, aged forty-five to fifty-five, from all socio-economic levels.

A woman who is perimenopausal but doesn't know it goes to her doctor to report heavy bleeding. 'Is this the Change?' she asks. He tells her she's too young for the Change, but she'd better have a D&C. The study investigators follow up eighteen months later. By now, the woman has gone in for two or three D&Cs, which haven't stopped the bleeding because it wasn't pathology. It was normal perimenopause. But by now the woman is so scared, she ends up having a hysterectomy which wasn't necessary, and which only serves to bring on menopause sooner and with far more severe symptoms.

Now, what could this woman have done instead? A simple office biopsy of the lining of the uterus could document any evidence of pre-malignant changes. Or, she could have a hysteroscopy, an examination that allows the physician to look inside the cavity of the uterus and see if there is a polyp. If there is still doubt, she could take a three-month course of hormone replacement, to see if the dysfunctional bleeding is resolved.

Some women with fibroid tumours do have clear indicators for hysterectomy: first, rapid growth of the tumour which may be a sign of cancer developing in the fibroid; second, uncontrollable bleeding; third, fibroid size so large that other organs may be compromised; or, finally, intractable pain.

Educated women, particularly in the United States, are beginning to see themselves as selective consumers of health care and refusing to accept any doctor's word as oracular. And when they find out how little the doctors know, or anybody knows, about this oldest of female physical transitions, they are mad as hell.

The TV producer who suffered embarrassment with hot flushes at a dinner party is a case in point. When she reported her problem to her gynaecologist, he said, noticeably bored, 'Oh, yeah, fifty years old, you're right on target. Menopause.'

'What can I do about it?' inquired the take-charge producer, accustomed to handling an eight-million-dollar budget.

'You just start taking oestrogen.'

She asked what were the implications of taking hormones.

'Well, you'll have to go for a breast X-ray twice a year instead of once a year. But there's no risk.'

'If there's no risk, then why do I have to go twice as often?' she replied, thinking logically. He brushed off her question with a few remarks that sounded like he was reading out of a manual: *How to Handle The Over-the-Hill Patient.*

'That made me defiant,' says the producer. Finally she insisted he tell her if there was anything that would treat the hot flushes. He told her about the old standby called Bellergal. He warned, 'But that won't help with irritability, depression, crying – all the rest of it.'

'Maybe I won't have any "rest of it",' the producer said, her adrenaline pumping full strength. 'In the meantime, so I don't have to spend the next ten years in a terrycloth robe, I'll try the Bellergal.' She got up to leave.

'You can do that,' said the gynaecologist, with what she read as an arrogant smirk. 'But you'll be back.'

The normal preamble to menopause is sometimes treated with a casualness bordering on the criminal. 'This uterus looks a little bit tired,' a male gynaecologist told a forty-year-old North Carolina woman, 'guess we'll take her out.' It was typical of the attitude among some doctors that the uterus is little more than a nuisance. Since this patient was a housekeeper, without all the fancy scientific words to defend the tired 'her', all she could do was 'fight to keep my uterus'.

At some level we *know* when the Change begins to come upon us. The sense of unease or disequilibrium is something women feel, though it remains incomprehensible to those who have not experienced it. Isn't it amazing that women should allow organized medicine, filtered through a male perspective, to tell us how we feel? (How many men know what it's like to be one week late? Or two weeks early while you're teaching a class in a white suit?) Medical breakthroughs in this century have given us the gift of greatly extended life spans; now attention should be turned to bringing *healthier* life spans. And that means women must become informed, active consumers of good health care. But because up to the present day we have accepted a way of thinking that denies or denigrates this epic change in our bodies and the exciting new vistas it can open in our minds, we have failed to demand that decent scientific research be done.

In America, our tax dollars have supported massive research into heart disease among men (while leaving women out of those clinical trials entirely), but our national health institutes cannot give us any definitive data about the long-term impact of the body's post-reproductive state on women's health. The NIH has spared only 13 percent of its revenues to study women's health. In Britain, the National Osteoporosis Society launched a major GP campaign in January 1993. The Society has been working for two years with the Department of Health and the Royal College of GPs to produce a pack for GPs and nurse practitioners, to be sent free to every GP practice in the UK (about twelve thousand in all).

If you compare the level of our scientific knowledge about the causes and effects of menopause with the evolution of modern medicine, it is as though bacteria have not been discovered yet and we are still dependent on leeches and roots and shamans to cure what ails us.

Medical schools still use terms such as *the weeping of the uterus* to describe menstruation, assigning emotions to a bodily organ because it wasn't fertilized by male sperm that month. The classical medical terminology for menopause is *ovarian failure*.

Another way of seeing it would be as *ovarian fulfilment*. One has put in thirty or forty years of ripening eggs and enduring the hormonal mischief of monthly cycles, on the chance another child is wanted. Enough, say most women in middle age. We're ready to move on now, to find our place in the world, free of the responsibilities of our procreative years. It's time to take risks and pursue passions and allow ourselves adventures perhaps set aside way back at thirteen, when we accepted the cultural script for our gender that denied those dreams. It's time to play! And kick up some dust!

CINDERELLA
HITS MENOPAUSE

As the pacesetters among baby boom generation women discover menopause on their horizon, they will bring it out of the closet. It has been happening only in the last year, beginning with conversations that in a previous generation would have been unimaginable.

I went to Los Angeles to join in such conversations. It seems that my article had stirred up a little *frisson* of fright among some of the movers and shakers in the film community. In that world, where leading ladies never look a day over twenty-nine and studio executives start subtracting years from their résumés before they hit thirty, Hollywood producer Lynda Guber had picked up a copy of *Vanity Fair* and discovered a cloud on the horizon of her perfect existence.

'*Menopause!*' she shrieked. 'God, I've never seen that word written.'

Lynda is a sizzling redhead from Brooklyn who has reached the pinnacle of Hollywood society together with her husband, Peter Guber, producer of *Batman* and *Rainman* and now the head of SONY Pictures Entertainment. The next day she bumped into Joanna Poitier at a Beverly Hills bistro and asked innocently, 'How are you doing?'

'I'm a lunatic, I'm going through menopause and empty nest at the same time,' said the beautiful actress-wife of actor Sidney Poitier. (It is culture-specific to Hollywood to identify women by their husbands' professional status).

This is fantastic, thought Lynda. *This woman is ready to talk about how she feels.* Lynda herself had already decided 'the impact of menopause will not be devastating on me, that's what my holistic belief system tells me'; but all she knew about it, in fact, was that the subject was a real no-no. Lynda is committed to being a consciousness-raiser of people in the movie business, having co-founded an organization, Education First!, that spreads positive messages through TV shows. She passed the word to a friend, Annie Gilbar, editor of *LA Style*. 'Annie, I have an idea. I'd like to have a meeting on menopause with the girls.' The first invitees backed off. But word spread, and before long it became such a cachet event there had to be a luncheon and a dinner group. I was invited to come out and speak to both.

Going to Hollywood to talk about menopause was a little bit like going to Las Vegas to sell savings accounts. Such is the fetish over youthfulness in Southern California, one half expects there to be an ordinance against menopause there. 'Women who are menopausal in California are around the bend – they view it like cancer,' I was warned by a Chinese medicine specialist with a deluxe and desperate clientele in Los Angeles.

Nevertheless, it was a golden opportunity. California women in the boomer vanguard are normally the most uninhibited among their species in speaking out about whatever bothers them. I quickly discovered, however, that even they – women who have access to the most up-to-date information, women who are religious about doing the stations of their Nautilus machines, women who have phone indexes of dozens of doctors, not to mention the best acupuncturists, herbalists, liposuctionists, and shrinks – *even they* didn't have any answers on menopause. In fact, they had never discussed the questions, even among themselves. When they did come together to confront the subject, they reflected many of the secret fears and defensive reactions common among women everywhere.

Lynda invited us to gather at her Japanese-style fantasy beach house. At the door each woman was invited to leave her shoes on a shelf and choose a kimono. I kept looking for a grey hair in the crowd – scarcely a one among this mostly blonde, mostly mid-fortyish group. The guests draped themselves over big black chenille cushions on tansu boxes in the screening room. The stage was set. It was reminiscent of slumber parties in junior high school, when girls played dress-up and talked about taboo subjects like sex. But now we were grownups; the very fact they had showed up was, in this subculture, an act of bravery.

'I invited Glenn Close to come,' said one of the women. 'I thought she was going to faint dead away.'

I began by asking those present to introduce themselves, give their age, and say why they had come – what meaning did menopause have for them? The wife of one of the town's top studio executives confessed she usually shunned 'negative subjects', but her mother was dead and she had no one else to consult. The head of her own executive search firm described herself as an information junkie. 'My gynaecologist tells me that I'm not going through the Change at all, but I know my body and I feel different over the past year. I've had occasional night sweats. I used to think I had a virus.'

Lisa Specht, a lawyer who is seen as the legal correspondent on ABC-TV's *Home Show*, has no children and said she didn't think she had to worry about menopause, at least until she was fifty-five or something. 'I haven't had any symptoms yet, except that my skin has been oily,' she assured herself.

The outspoken Joanna Poitier broke the ice. She was willing to admit she might be going through menopause, although her primary concern was letting go of her two daughters, now eighteen and twenty. 'I keep waking up in the middle of the night, changing my nightgown. I went to the gynaecologist, and she told me that I was still moist. She said I won't probably go into menopause for another two years. I have night sweats. I tried it without the duvet and the nightgown, and I still have night sweats. I have day sweats too! The back of my neck is damp all day long.'

The next speaker was immediately recognizable. Lesley Ann Warren, the movie actress we all remember from her ethereal portrayal of Cinderella in the TV musical, is even more beautiful today. Her features are still delicate, her body is still slim and supple, and reddish brown hair ripples over her shoulders.

More appealing than all that is the quickened intelligence and candour that she has earned over forty years and brought to her more recent roles in the films *Victor/Victoria*, and *Choose Me*. But Lesley Ann makes her living here in Cinderella Land, where girls are never supposed to grow up. Hollywood ruthlessly cuts the finest actresses once they reach forty – yes, even Meryl! Studio executives will callously describe a 38-year-old actress who is still gorgeous as 'Over the hill', or 'She's an old hag'. As an actress in that workplace, Lesley Ann Warren is torn between her liberated feminist beliefs and the devastating reality that every day her worth is judged by her age and her looks.

Divorced from Jon Peters, former co-head of the former Columbia Studios, with whom she had a son, Lesley Ann has been single for some time. She now has a new love. It was he who found a xeroxed copy of my *Vanity Fair* article lying around. Lesley Ann wanted to educate herself on the subject before it happened so she could deal with it homeopathically and herbally, as she does everything else. She had forgotten to hide the evidence.

'You know, I read this article,' he said casually one night. *Omigod, he's found me out!* was the actress's first thought. 'I was really scared he would think *I* was menopausal. I felt ashamed.' But he surprised her.

'I'm glad I read it. I feel like any man who's in a relationship with a woman dealing with this must be very loving, very aware, and very present,' he said.

Lesley Ann counted her new love among an ultramicroscopic subspecies of the male genus, at least as they are bred by the movie business. 'In all the rest of my experience, men are so staggeringly uneducated in this area, it's deadly for us,' she told the group. 'Most men I know run from the word *menopause*.'

'We're afraid to educate the men, that's our problem,' amended Joanna. 'I have never been afraid to say how old I am. I've never had surgery or collagen or anything like that. And I don't feel any less terrific because I'm menopausal. Whoever you are with, they should experience the whole thing that you're experiencing.' Joanna added vociferously, 'I take no aspirin, no Tylenol, if I have a headache, I live through it. I don't believe in pills. I know that I will not take hormones, because to me it's unnatural.'

The word *holistic* was almost a fetish in this group. Used indiscriminately, it might mean one who never uses Tylenol, or one who has stopped taking drugs and alcohol, or one who consults Chinese medical doctors and herbalists but *never* a member of the American Medical Association (AMA). A bouncy talent agent with a blonde boy-cut admitted she was taking hormones; *admitted*, because, like so many women, her decision was tinged with guilt. 'I knew something was up when I went to a restaurant and had to ask the waiter for two menus – one to see what I was ordering and the other to fan myself.'

Knowing laughter rippled through the group. We decided that if we met again we would call ourselves The Fan Club.

The agent revealed a more intimate reason for her decision. 'One night when my husband and I were having sex, it felt like I was a virgin. I said, "Something is wrong here". My gynaecologist took a blood test and told me it was the Change of Life.' She emphasized that she was on a very low dose of hormone replacement therapy, and that she was happy with the results.

Joanna Poitier broke in with a question on everybody's mind. 'Is it okay to go through the rest of life without oestrogen?'

Dr Allen said there was no definitive answer. 'When we are in this part of our lives, we have to make decisions about what it is that we want. Beyond the symptomatic discomforts, there are also medical issues that bear on our long-term health – osteoporosis, heart disease, breast and uterine cancer.' Dr Allen's advice was to gather as much information as possible, including about one's own family history, to find out if there is a medical reason to take hormone replacement therapy, and then make a decision.

'But we don't have to make a decision for life. We make a decision for three months, and then we make a decision again,' she added, sowing visible relief in some of the tense faces. Others were impatient with this answer. They had come looking for a risk-free, all-natural curative.

Mary Miccuci introduced herself as a 'stress queen'. A tall, Cher-like streak of a woman who started her own catering business, Along Came Mary, she dashes around Hollywood putting on spreads for the stars. Her signs of menopause began with palpitations; she thought she was having a heart attack. 'The quality of my life is changing – all of our lives are changing. I want information!' she said angrily, pitching forward to lean her elbows on her knees. 'I want to go through this process as quickly as possible. I'm on a holistic journey to deal with it. Are there the right herbs to take care of the silent killers – heart disease and osteoporosis?'

Surely what they all wanted to hear from me and Dr Allen was that some magic regimen – yoga and yogurt, or yams and ginseng and green leafy vegetables – would allow them to remain as middle-aged women exactly as they had been: youthful wives, sexually appealing and responsive lovers, efficient career builders. They were not yet ready to consider a new self-definition. And until one is ready, the information that is available is not much use.

'I think that we have all been too passive about what the outcome of our lives should be,' Mary continued huffily. 'Because I tell you, the way I felt for a year was pretty shitty. I have a five-and-a-half-year-old little girl, and I want to be so together for this kid. This menopause stuff, I'll be goddamned if I'll let it get in my way.'

Mary's hostility towards the whole subject was revelatory. She had become accustomed to managing her life like a man, according to goals, timetables, balance sheets. She is a businesswoman accustomed to efficiency; in fact, she had to leave early to cater a screening party for Bette Midler's newest film. But now, at the peak of her productivity, she is feeling violated by this reassertion of her body's biologic identity. There is nothing efficient about 'this menopause stuff'.

Aloma Ichinose, a photographer equally active in her career, had taken the opposite approach. 'I'm going through the

Change right now. I feel great about it. But at first it was a nightmare. I was raised by a man so none of this was ever talked about.' Allowing time for trial and error, Aloma had made several different decisions over the previous year. When urine and blood tests confirmed that she was in menopause, her doctor put her on Premarin. To her, it felt like doing drugs. 'I did the Premarin for six months. I felt wonderful, and all my symptoms – the disrupted sleep, the forgetfulness —went away.' She added defensively, 'I'm not into drugs. I haven't had a drink in years. But I was really worried about bone loss. I'm active, I'm a photographer, I need my strength.' Eventually, the fear and guilt over taking hormones got to her, and after the six months she stopped. 'And all the symptoms returned,' she admitted. 'I just didn't feel well, and so I'm back on it again and I feel good.'

An art gallery owner pressed the issue of age-prevention. 'How long do you take this? Will it prolong our youth? We are young in our forties, where people of other generations weren't. I'm forty-seven years old, but I don't think that I am forty-seven in numbers. I have the same energy as always.'

Joanna, whose blonde tendrils and soft curves help her to maintain the jolly all-American-girl good looks of a perpetual cheerleader, is able to maintain the illusion of her inner eye: 'I still feel like I'm twenty-eight. I wear my hair the same way, I'm twenty-eight years old.'

Another woman in the room muttered, 'But you're not. And they *know* you're not.'

It cut like a flesh wound into the self-image of every woman there. They were all attractive, and that statement didn't even need the qualifying prefix 'still'. External beauty wasn't the real problem. It was the dysynchrony between their idealized inner image – the woman they were at their nubile peak – and blanks where the faces and bodies and spirits of their future selves would have to be filled in, sooner or later. As vanguard baby boomers, they agreed, they belonged to the most pampered, narcissistic and obstinately adolescent generation in American history. 'We have delayed duty, responsibility and commitment,' wrote a spokeswoman for their generation,

Lynn Smith, in the *Los Angeles Times*. 'We have dieted, jogged, and exercised so much, we look and actually *think* we are five to ten years younger than we are.'

The most telling reaction of all came from a sleek-looking South African woman who had been mute all night. Before I left, she took me aside and asked the quintessential Southern California question:

'Tell me, what can I do so I *don't have to have this?*'

BOOMERS'
GIFT TO WOMEN

As a woman looks ahead to the Change, it is natural to focus entirely on the loss of powers one has taken for granted in previous stages. The youthful looks you could always trade on, and the magical powers of procreation that connected you to the cycle of all life – these are the God-given, gloriously unfair advantages of being born a well-formed woman. Suddenly, in the mid-forties, one must face the fact that these powers are ebbing. What will replace them?

The women who attended the luncheon meeting in Beverly Hills were ready to confront such issues. It was a mix of professionals who had left a mark on their respective fields: a top state politician, a mayor, and a judge were interspersed with well-known screenwriters, entertainment producers, and social activists. All but three of those present were in their mid-forties with still-young children.

'So many of us know each other,' Annie Gilbar kept remarking, 'and we talk about a lot of things – children, sex, everything – but this subject has never come up. Not once.'

Two of the creative talents in today's film industry were among the group: Meg Kasdan, co-screenwriter with husband

Lawrence Kasdan of *Grand Canyon*, and executive producer Carole Isenberg (*The Color Purple* and *This Is My Life*). Both were flabbergasted when they couldn't think of a single reference in a film to a woman going through the Change and the impact it had on her life. 'I'm always sneaking messages in about women's lives, but never this,' said Carole. 'It's a sorry statement that shows how unwilling and uncomfortable we have been to deal with this issue.' Meg added, 'Mature women – that is, over forty – are almost invisible in Hollywood movies.'

Once people began to talk about menopause as more than a matter of spigots and pipes and secretions involving our organs, an important issue surfaced. Losing the magic – that was the deeper mutation to be accepted. The graduation from our fertile years resonates in our psyches as deeply as the squirm and throb in the belly of first pregnancy signifies our awesome powers of creation. Like most graduations, it is the occasion for both relief and sadness.

'For many of us who waited until we were well into our thirties and even early forties before having children, the physical power of giving birth is still palpable – it touches something very deep and instinctual,' ventured Suzanne Rosenblatt Buhai, a psychotherapist. 'That flame of the instinctual being extinguished is not as readily dealt with as one might think.'

Dealing with loss is one of the tasks we struggle with in every passage, but it is particularly poignant as women notice the first skips in a fertility we have probably taken for granted. The feelings were brought out by a woman who has obviously delighted in maternity. Joyce Bogart Trabulus has two children and a quartet of stepchildren in her life, and is further fulfilled by community caretaking in the form of running charities for cancer and AIDS research. She has no desire to have any more children. No *daylight world* desire.

'And yet I really feel sadness every time I think about it,' she admitted. 'I was forty-one when I had my last child, who's three years old now – I almost feel like a grandmother to my own kid. And I sometimes catch myself thinking, *Oh god, this is fabulous, I'd love to do this again.* It's a great loss to know that it will be impossible for me. It's not like I want another one. And I'm not menopausal, or even pre-menopausal. But I look at a baby and say, "Oh".'

Suzanne mused out loud, 'Given our generational narcissism – whether it's because of our sheer numbers, Dr Spock, or the dominant influence of psychoanalysis – I just wonder if this concern with self is now being focused on menopause. Are we getting all worked up over something that is in fact quite normal and has been experienced since time immemorial? Perhaps the best gift we can give society at this stage is to see this as something very positive. If we can normalize this experience, as Gail says, it will help women deal with it. Otherwise, women will take on the responsibility of this somehow being their fault – they are supposed to be pulling out of this funk.'

One of the few women in the room over fifty, Vicki Reynolds, mayor of Beverly Hills, looked around the group with eagerness and some envy. 'I am almost a generation ahead of most of you,' she said. 'I have seen women my age go through menopause without the benefit of any medical enlightenment – ignorant of all you have been saying. Now we look to you, the baby boom generation, to talk about this openly and explore the effects and benefits of menopause. That's so exciting.'

It was agreed that the vestigial attitude surrounding menopause – 'I'm no good any more' – would be changed by the way women like themselves handled it. I suggested, only half-seriously, 'If every woman in menopause told five people in the next week, those five people would have an entirely different view of it. "This dish is in menopause? Well, maybe it isn't so terrible."'

Dr Allen observed that at this stage we have responsibilities to the world, not just to our tiny communities. She is excited every day by finding new channels to educate women about their bodies. 'That's my public passion,' she said. 'But we also need something for ourselves – new passions all the time.'

I added wickedly, 'And they may include a 25-year-old lover.'

'Yeah, a *blind* twenty-five-year-old lover!' amended one of the California women.

With a whooping and shimmying of laughter, the session ended. Seventeen women went out into the world to resume their balancing acts between careers, husbands, children, car pools, social and spiritual life, too busy to worry much about menopause, but better prepared for the future. Laughter and forgetting ... two of the best gifts women of any age can share with one another.

But something hopeful, something even incendiary had come out of those two sessions with California women. Their need to know was beginning to overcome their fear of knowing. It convinced me that the pacesetting women of this generation will shift the boundaries as well as the meaning of menopause: they will redefine it, and *live it*, as a mid-life experience of minor importance in the scheme of a long and lushly various life.

THE 'WHAT ABOUT ME?' SYNDROME

Less privileged women often assume that menopause is just another burden of being a woman and simply bear it, though not grinning. But the class differences are glaring. The population tapped for the rare studies has been almost exclusively white, well-educated and motivated to take care of their health preventively. The vast majority of women in lower socio-economic groups have no idea of the long-term health issues related to 'the Change'. They are so accustomed to bleeding and having cramps and premenstrual tension that when they hit menopause they just shrug and say, 'Here we go again – male doctors treating me like I don't matter a damn.'

That was Kate McNally's first reaction. A secretarial assistant in local government in a medium-size Long Island town, she is now fifty-four. All her life Kate has been a great coper, having had four children close together and launched them all as young adults of whom she can be proud. Her reward? 'The most frustrating phase I've ever been through in my life – it's horrendous! I've never felt so helpless. Nobody understands menopause. And nobody knows what to do about it.'

Kate went to her gynaecologist complaining of heavy bleeding. After a questionable Pap smear, a cone biopsy was done followed by a D&C. She was put on oestrogen and told to have a mammogram. The results weren't conveyed to her for two months. A lump had been found. Of course, at first she blamed the hormones. But the great majority of breast tumours, including hers, are slow-growing. Her disease had probably been developing, undetected, for several years. The irony is, many women do not bother with a mammogram *until* they consult a doctor about indications of menopause. If a tumour is found, the culprit may look like hormones, but is probably the result of more careful medical surveillance.

After two lumpectomies, Kate is off oestrogen for ever and bedevilled by menopausal symptoms no one can tell her how to relieve. 'I feel betrayed,' she says softly. 'I've always put others before myself. By this age I have more money to work with and more leisure time with the kids gone. I should have the energy to do the things I've always wanted.' I asked what things she had looked forward to.

'Getting a decent night's sleep.' The modest expectation is betrayed by the dull film over her blue eyes. 'You go for years with little babies waking you up all night. Then the teen years when you can't sleep for worrying because they're out in your car. And now *I'm* the one awake all night!' She laughs hard. Her husband seems wonderfully supportive, and Kate is determined to cope with this stage as she has with other trials in the past. But after months of sleep deprivation, no wonder Kate, like so many menopausal women, says she feels frustrated.

Her sister, Bindy, is only forty-two and very attractive, with long, curly red hair and a sugar-doughnut figure wrapped in shorts and a T-shirt, but already she is wrestling with the emotional preamble to menopause. 'I used to be the no-worry type: just leave the house, go to the beach – nothing ever bothered me,' she says. 'I lost my temper but once in a blue moon.' Now, she's a virtual powder keg. When her son didn't come to the table until his dinner was cold, she jumped up in such a childish rage she knocked over a chair. 'Everybody looked at me as if I had three heads.'

She told her girlfriend later, 'They measured the chemicals in my brain with a blood test. They said the chemical was out of balance and that indicated I was in menopause.'

'That explains why you're so moody,' sympathized her friend.

'Moody! I'm not moody!' Bindy remembers shrieking. 'How can you say that? You're my best friend!'

These powerful hormones do, in fact, cross the blood–brain bridge. Sensors in the brain that control emotions pick up a signal when there is an erratic production of either oestrogen or progesterone. In a person whose nervous system is finely tuned, these sensors overreact, triggering brain-chemistry changes and emotional symptoms. Veteran gynaecologists affirm that some women can have physical symptoms from even slight changes in the amount of oestrogen produced.

Every morning, as a waitress in a busy coffee shop, Bindy has to stroke hundreds of people who haven't had coffee yet. 'The doctor told me to stop smoking, cut down on cholesterol, and avoid stress. Ha, avoid stress! How?'

She knows she is being grouchy and impossible. 'But I can't control it. And I'm afraid if I take this oestrogen, then I'll have lumps like my sister.'

Women like Kate and Bindy are often caught in the middle between caring for ageing, fragile parents and dealing with the lingering financial dependence of children. Many experience the 'What about me?' syndrome. They are not accustomed to nurturing themselves. But even as they are encouraged by books like this to pamper themselves through this transition, Western society is making more demands on them today than ever. Most middle-aged Americans today still have living parents, a change in family dynamics with no precedent in history. With many more people in the US and Europe living into their eighties and nineties, and fewer children per family, geriatric researchers warn that almost every woman is going to have to take care of an ageing parent or parent-in-law.

That will put more and more women on 'the daughter track', possibly for a decade or more, just as they are emerging from the 'mummy track'. Traditionally, it has been middle-aged women who are depended upon to do the work of unpaid caregiving for the disabled elderly at home. But women now also fill nearly half the paid positions *outside* the home. At just the stage when they expect to enter the most focused and productive period of their working lives, with their children grown and gone, they may not be able to carry the new double burden of elder-caregiving and full-time career. Many will have to switch to part-time jobs, forfeit promotions, or quit their jobs altogether, unless they demand reforms in public policy and decent elder-care. The cruel choice for a growing number of menopausal-aged women will be: Do I take care of my mother in her old age, or provide for independence in my own old age?

No wonder, just beneath the calm, composed surface of many middle-aged women, one finds fears of being invisible, dependent and, finally, decrepit.

ACROSS COLOUR, CLASS AND CULTURE LINES

The chief reason for the silence and apprehension surrounding the subject of menopause in American society is our phobia about ageing. Cross-cultural studies of women and menopause reveal that the Change of Life is experienced differently depending on one's cultural assumptions about ageing, femininity, and the societal role of the older woman. When the American sociologist Pauline Bart studied anthropological accounts of the status of women in a large number of cultures, she found that the feminine role assumed by a woman in her fertile years was in all cultures reversed after menopause.

Anthropologist Mary Catherine Bateson points out: 'In many societies women are granted a greater degree of freedom after menopause than they were permitted in their reproductive years. This may be because women no longer represent a risk of "pollution", or no longer need to be sequestered as sex objects through whom their husbands might be dishonoured.' Indian women of the Rajput caste do not complain of depression or psychological symptoms of menopause since they are freed from veiled invisibility and at last are able to sit and joke with the men, reports anthropologist Marcha Flint. Furthermore, in some traditional societies, such as Iran's, women only come into their own when they have an adult son. Bateson describes how grown-up sons literally pay court to their mothers, visiting them with news and flowers.

Women in Asian countries report fewer and less severe symptoms than menopausal women in the West – even though the mean age at menopause is the same across the board (slightly over fifty-one years). These findings were presented at the Sixth International Congress on the Menopause, held in Bangkok in late 1990. The study included women from Hong Kong, Malaysia, the Philippines, South Korea, Taiwan, Indonesia, and Singapore.

In China, where age is venerated, menopausal symptoms are rarely reported. Similarly, anthropologist Margaret Lock observed after studying a thousand Japanese women that 65 percent of them consider menopause uneventful. The Japanese language does not even have a word for hot flushes. (A report in *The Lancet*, however, describes 'sinking spells' among Japanese women, rather like the swooning of Victorian women.) However, the virtual non-existence of hot flushes in

Japanese women is *not cultural,* according to Locke. It is due primarily to their different diet and the vigorous physical exercise built into the life of even elderly Japanese women. Their blood streams show high levels of soy (a source of oestrogen) and calcium from a fish-dominated diet. And because most Japanese women have small kitchens, they walk or bike daily to the shops and hand-carry groceries back home, routinely enjoying a much higher degree of exercise than most middle-class women undertake in the West. As a result, menopausal women in Japan are not as prone to menopausal health problems as Western women; they have a much lower incidence of heart disease, osteoporosis and breast cancer. Although only 2 percent of Japanese women take hormones, they are the longest living women in the world.

In America, youth and desirability go hand in hand, and the role for the older woman is uncertain at best. Ours is also an overweight, underexercised culture, particularly in the upper age brackets. Very few roles or jobs in the information age demand that American women over forty exert much more physical effort than opening their car doors and microwaves. But although menopause in the US is defined primarily in hormonal terms, cultural attitudes do cut deeply, casting the signs and symptoms in a negative light. Of two thousand five hundred Massachusetts women aged forty-five to fifty-five studied by Harvard sociologist John McKinlay and epidemiologist Sonja McKinlay, most anticipated menopause with relief. But, for those whose self-worth rests primarily in appearance and sexual desirability, passing fifty is like *taking the veil*; suddenly they feel invisible.

Although I did not undertake a 'scientific' sampling of American women's menopausal experiences, I did interview well over a hundred women from diverse racial, class, and educational backgrounds. I discovered that the women who enjoy a boost in post-menopausal status and self-esteem are those who perform roles in which intellect, judgement, creativity, or spiritual strength is primarily valued – politicians, educators, law-makers, doctors, nurse-supervisors, therapists, writers, artists, clergywomen, etc. – while women whose worth was earlier judged primarily on their looks and sex appeal – movie actresses, performers, many full-time wives and mothers – are diminished in status. We know that middle-class housewives who are over-involved with their children are the most likely to suffer depression in this stage of life. But they, too, are able to change stale self-images if they are willing to leave the comfort of familiarity and take the risk of starting a new direction in their Second Adulthood. Women who build close bonds to grandchildren may make themselves indispensable, and often enjoy a tender and playful intimacy that brings them closer than they were to their own children.

Black women in general are more likely than white women to pass through menopause with no psychological problems. Why? I wondered. After the book was published, a friend and former professor of adult development, Clementine Pugh, gathered together a fascinating discussion group with twenty accomplished African-American women, most of them educators with advanced degrees. They agreed that black women do not measure their femininity and sensuality only by how they look. Nor is their self-worth attached to their age – how young they look. A great deal of a black woman's sexuality is defined by her spiritual strength, a strength dictated by her historical situation.

Middle-class black women come out of matrilineal tradition. Never having been pampered by life or put on a pedestal while they were young, as white women are, they gain in prestige and self-esteem as they enter middle age. And they definitely *do not* give up on themselves as sexually desirable or desirous. What's more, sensuality, for the black woman, is not related to the European-American anorexic body type. Stop and think about the many great older black women entertainers who sing and shake and bring the house down – from Moms Mabley and Ma Rainey to Della Reese, Patti Labelle, and even the opera superstar Jesse Norman. The older and broader they are, it seems, the more shamelessly lusty they can be. In short, menopause is more readily accepted as an integral part of life.

In Britain, class strongly determines the menopausal experience (as does race in the US). Middle-class women today tend to be more open and willing to talk about menopause and to seek out a Well Woman clinic in one of the major cities; working-class women, who are generally more reticent and inhibited to begin with, aren't likely to ask many questions unless they run into real medical problems. If they go to their GP with the usual vague constellation of symptoms, they'll likely be told, 'It's just your age, dear.'

Facts of British life, like retirement age and pension benefits, foster even crueller stereotypes about older women than in the States. 'There are few role models for women of my generation in the office,' laments Eve Pollard. Having attained a position of power and high profile in the media, the controversial London editor believes she takes a great deal of nasty flak because women who are successful in Britain are denigrated. 'Whereas men grey at the temples, and move effortlessly up to the top jobs, when I'm wrinkled and older looking, they'll probably say, "What does she know? She's an old lady."'

Many of the successful professional women in the City, according to those I interviewed, are turning to hormone replacement therapy in hopes of minimizing the penalties of age stereotyping on their careers. But there are many other equally intelligent and accomplished British women who resent male experts and commercial drug companies herding them towards chemical dependency, like fertility impersonators. Some already feel so marked down as middle-aged women, they take the attitude, *Why bother?* I visited such a woman in London.

It's a Saturday night, and it probably would have been a lonely one for the researcher if I hadn't come by to talk about her report on ageing in the United Kingdom. Jane I'll call her, since she doesn't like to personalize; she remains the expert, at arm's length from her results. Jane lives in an Edwardian terraced house on a genteel square in Southwest London. She and her husband bought it in the Sixties and had small children here, renting the top floors to pay for it. Its walls are steeped in sweet memories for her. The great white shutters guarding her tall windows are rolled back, filling the front room with bronzed late-afternoon sun filtered through lacy acacia trees. Time seems to stand still, as if she lives in a drawing room from a different century.

In fact, Jane is a dynamic woman in her fifties who broke new ground in negotiating a 'top girl' position for herself in the civil service. Making no concession to vanity, she goes without makeup and keeps her grey hair chopped in Joan of Arc-style severity. Just as she was about to deliver her crowning achievement, a major national study on ageing, she developed back spasms. She ignored the problem until something went in the connection between her spine and hip. Laid flat, she is forced to write her final reports while lying face down on a foam mattress on the living room floor. It's the only way she can manage.

Now she lies on her side, Cleopatra-style, with a glass of white wine, and talks intelligently and crisply about the emerging poverty class of older women. 'We have got to the point now where a couple who reaches the age of fifty has almost a 50 percent chance they will both be alive at the age of seventy-five,' she says. 'That's the good news. But the breakup of marriages among couples in their fifties is an increasing phenomenon.'

Who usually initiates the divorce? I ask.

'Usually the man goes off with a younger woman.' The husband's occupational pension belongs to him, she explains, and if the woman has not had a career and earned a pension in her own right, all she is entitled to is the paltry state pension given to single people. The long-standing wife loses her husband's death benefit, too. 'The second wife picks up the widow's benefit, and because she's younger, she lives longer,' says Jane. So pervasive is the phenomenon, insurance companies are re-costing the contributions necessary to cover widow's benefits on the *probability* that husbands today will leave their original spouse and remarry a younger woman. So there she is, codified in the actuarial figures: the wife dumped in the middle of life.

'An enormous number of those women will face poverty,' Jane sums up in a monotone.

Why aren't British women making a fuss about this? I wonder aloud.

Jane says she doesn't think they realize what is happening.

Perhaps, I suggest, already feeling marked down as a menopausal woman, they don't feel they have any right to make a fuss.

'There is a real problem for an awful lot of women in this country,' Jane acknowledges. 'If they have been dumped, or even widowed, there is a lack of feeling of self-worth. If the marriage ends, for whatever reason, having a sense of identity with which to survive is a big problem.' She winces as she moves slightly. 'I suppose it's the equivalent of a bloke losing his job. In our generation the woman's identity is entirely bound up with the marriage and children, and the man's is entirely bound up with his job.'

I ask if her studies show any link between increasing male redundancy and sexual dysfunction. The question seems to take her by surprise. 'I have seen nothing in all the literature that links sexual behaviour with economic change,' Jane says. 'It's not been documented. That, in itself, is interesting.' I propose some possible connections: a man who loses his job, irrevocably, suffers from lowered self-esteem. Let's say, at the same time, his wife enters menopause and feels her self-worth precarious, since she's no longer fertile and her kids no longer need her. She doesn't have any severe medical problems, so she hasn't been motivated to seek homeopathic remedies or HRT for her menopausal state. Why bother? she says. For her, sexual desire has waned. For him, sexual potency must be reproven. He's desperate to demonstrate that he still matters in the world, so he rushes out to find the novelty of a younger woman to restore his erections. Wife #1 is dumped, thereby confirming her shattered self-esteem. End of story.

'Isn't the sociological deck stacked against mid-life marriages surviving?' I ponder. 'What's to keep them together?'

Jane draws a long breath. It's an interesting question, she says. Her own inquiry does not feed into a personal life cycle perspective, she adds. But recently, something like this has happened to her. After thirty years of happy, fruitful marriage, her husband upped and left. One gets the sense of a life that has been truncated.

With difficulty, Jane treads lightly around identifying with the emotionally and financially deprived class of discarded wives. 'Most women don't have either the social or the financial security,' she says. 'I've got both, but I've become very conscious of what it would be like if I were going through this without that inner security. I suspect that more American women have that security than here, because we're much more polarized in male-female roles in my generation in Britain.'

Jane's sadness begins to colour her otherwise stoutly professional voice. She has allowed her horizons to begin shrinking. 'Outside cosmopolitan London, if you're a woman on your own, you tend no longer to be asked to parties and social functions of couples,' she complains, 'because you're always assumed to be after somebody else's husband.'

Even in London, yes, right around the corner, at the neighbourhood restaurant she used to frequent with her husband, the whole social chemistry changed the first time she appeared without a man. 'Will somebody else be joining you?' insisted the waiter more than once, making it clear he found it unseemly for two women to be dining together. Finally, cutting with chilly politesse, he said, 'Now *ladies*, what can I do for you?' Anticipating the scorn and possible insolence of waiters, Jane has stopped going out with women friends in the evening. Even she, a woman who has been the boss of hundreds of people and presided over a multi-billion pound budget, is allowing social cues to redefine her as one of the invisible postmenopausal women.

Although she can rattle off the statistics that show the price paid for ignoring the possibility of osteoporosis, she hasn't shown any interest in getting a bone density test herself. As she lies flat on her back, she talks about a recent national fitness survey. 'The figures on people over fifty taking exercise here are terrible. We know now that walking, or some equivalent form of exercise for at least an hour a day, and aerobic exercise for twenty minutes twice a week, are the absolute minimum needed to keep up your stamina and suppleness.' She knows that the drastic decline in daily exercise among over-fifties Britons correlates with premature physical decline. 'Appropriate exercise can restore fitness, even at older ages,' she has learned. But Jane doesn't practise that either.

'Speaking personally, it's only if there's a real problem that you would go on to hormones. I haven't. *Why bother?*' Despite her own precarious physical condition, she has made a political decision.

'My own doctor is a left-wing radical lady,' she explains. 'Her view was that HRT is a conspiracy of men to keep women in a permanently pseudo-pregnant condition, and that one shouldn't go down this route.' In the next breath, Jane the researcher recounts new evidence that indicates that the worry over HRT raising the risk of breast cancer has been exaggerated. 'Doctors have done a review of the worldwide literature and find the risk of breast cancer, on the whole, is very slight,' she says, 'whereas the beneficial effect in protecting against heart disease is very much more substantial.' Still her attitude is, *Why bother?*

One who does bother, and very publicly, is Teresa Gorman. She commenced a new career as a Member of Parliament at the age of fifty-six. A vigorous and opinionated personality, with clear eyes and that English misted skin even a daughter might envy, the postmenopausal woman fibbed about her age. Her supporters were convinced she was a mere forty-seven. After winning the election with a comfortable majority, Gorman was caught out by a journalist. She decided to turn a mirror on the issue of age.

At a debate on women's health, the spunky new MP stood up and announced that she was ten years older than she had told her constituents. 'I'm fifty-six, heading up to sixty,' she said proudly. Shocked rigid, people were forced to confront their own age prejudices. Gorman let them know she'd used hormone therapy since she was fifty, and that she was still interesting to the man she'd married at nineteen.

Well, when the Essex MP introduced the taboo word 'menopause' into the snoozy male bastion of the House of Commons, it produced a shudder of embarrassment under the
port-wine-stained ties of her fellow parliamentarians. Some
walked out. Undaunted, dubbed by the media 'Saint Teresa of
the Menopause', Gorman enjoys being the most controversial
member of Parliament. She travels around the country telling
women that if they want to keep the older man from leaving
home for a dolly bird, they, too, will get smart and use HRT.
'If men had to put up with hot flushes and other symptoms of
the menopause,' she insists, 'treatment would be available
across the counter in Woolworth's.'

Gorman claims to have put HRT on the map in Britain. It
was she who started up the Amarant Trust to help women
obtain information about menopause. 'We now have our own
clinic and are the only organization in the UK that trains GPs
and health professionals,' she informed me.

Another reason for the fear inspired by the prospect of menopause is the assumption that it takes place at a single point in
time. 'Women are very frightened that at age forty-nine, all
these things they've read about – heart disease, osteoporosis,
vaginal atrophy – will happen all at once,' says Professor
Mansfield. 'No distinction is made between women's lives at
fifty and at seventy. We would never do this with men.'

It is important, then, to distinguish among the various
phases of the long menopausal passage. Archie Bunker probably spoke for many impatient husbands when he pressed his
long-suffering wife in a 1972 episode of *All in the Family*.

ARCHIE: Edith, if you're gonna have a Change of Life, you
gotta do it right now. I'm gonna give you just thirty
seconds. Now come on, CHANGE!
EDITH: Can I finish my soup first?

More changes probably take place during this passage than at
any other time in a woman's adult life. And as one moves
through the physical, psychological, social and spiritual
aspects of the transition, dramatic shifts in perspective occur.

There may be a transformation in the sense of time, of self in relation to others, and a rethinking of the negative vs. positive aspects of moving into a new and unfamiliar state of being.

The acute period of biological passage, or ovarian transition, spans five to seven years — usually forty-seven or forty-eight to the mid-fifties. But it is the beginning of a long and little-mapped stage of post-reproductive life. I propose three demarcations of this second adulthood for contemporary Western women: perimenopause (start of the transition); menopause (completion of the ovarian transition); and a stage I will call coalescence – the mirror image of adolescence – in which women can tap into the new vitality Margaret Mead called 'postmenopausal zest.'

The
Perimenopause
Panic

The earliest phase, perimenopause, is reminiscent of the first time one got one's period – the I-could-die feeling when a girlfriend whispered, 'You have a spot on the back of your skirt,' and you had to back out of the glee-club rehearsal so no one would see. And now, at the dignified apex of one's adulthood, to have to worry about being hit with surprise periods, hot flushes, night sweats, insomnia, incontinence, sudden bouts of waistline bloat, heart palpitations, crying for no reason, temper outbursts, migraines, itchy crawly skin, memory lapses – my God, what's going on?

It is during perimenopause – in their forties – that women feel most estranged from their bodies. The important thing to know is that for two to three years the female body is out of sync with its own chemistry.

Half of all women who have hot flushes will begin feeling them while they are still menstruating normally, starting as early as age forty. Studies show that most women have hot flushes for two years. One quarter of women have them for five years. And 10 percent have them for the rest of their lives.

The first sign of perimenopause, however, is very often *not* hot flushes, but gushing: a sudden heavy flow of blood that may be dark or clotted and that may seep through the normal protection. Dr Allen tells patients in their forties, 'Your cycle will get longer or shorter, lighter or heavier, closer together or farther apart. This is all normal.' She adds, 'Almost everybody bleeds erratically during perimenopause.'

(It happens when we stop ovulating every month. The months when ovulation doesn't occur, we produce no progesterone – the hormone ordinarily responsible for flushing the lining of the uterus. The endometrial lining becomes thicker and may not be entirely discarded until the next cycle, when the body deals with the previous buildup.)

One month a woman may have a heavy period, another month nothing; all of a sudden she may develop cysts in her breast, or functional ovarian cysts, and two months or a year later she may be back to normal. The reason for all the volatility is that hormone levels are surging and falling in frantic response to desperate signals from the brain to the pituitary. Her menstrual cycle not only becomes erratic, it is uncoupled from her temperature and sleep cycles, and affects her appetite, sexual interest, and overall sense of wellbeing. The body's whole balance is thrown off. While this can be very unsettling, it is *a temporary phenomenon*, and one should not be railroaded into a hysterectomy or on to hormones.

Phyllis Mansfield, the Penn State academic who spearheaded research on female cycles, registered the first signs of the Change in herself in her early forties. Having always had a normal and very predictable cycle, she was unnerved when her periods became heavier and more frequent. 'I would have to schedule family camping trips and conferences around my cycle.' Although she studied and went for checkups, still, in the back of her mind, was a common fear: *Are my organs deteriorating?*

She noticed something odd, too, about her moods. As a researcher, she knew that premenstrual stress occurs after ovulation. But when one's cycle becomes erratic, with periods every two or three weeks, or two or three months apart, how does one know when, or if, ovulation occurs?

'I'd have a really long period of magnificent energy and acute mental functioning, even brilliance, when I was never tired, always very up, producing like crazy. At first I thought, *Oh! so this is going to be part of my new personality*. Then just as suddenly I fell into a period of intense anxiety – and that lasted for a month. I thought, *So, is this it?* But once I got my period, the despond just lifted and dissipated in one day. So then you think, *What happens when there are no more cycles? Is there one mood that persists? Is it permanent mellowing? Permanent anything?*

What happens if I can't be me any more?

The vast majority of women have no idea they are in something called 'perimenopause'. Yet a woman's attitude and awareness going into this momentous passage has a profound impact on how it is experienced. As we know, the last person most women consult for information is a doctor. Those who do have often reached the point of panic.

'I think I'm going crazy' is a frequent frightened admission Dr Morris Notelovitz hears at the Women's Health Center in Gainesville, Florida. 'Many women feel it's very difficult to concentrate. They can hear what's going on, they know they're there, but it's as though their body is just witnessing.' These are the women whose hormones are falling and spiking and falling again, six times a day or even half a dozen times within an hour. They feel – and in fact they are – out of control of their bodies. They may also feel at the mercy of erratic moods. Is it all in their minds?

DANCING
AROUND
DEPRESSION

Whether or not depression is associated with menopause has been a subject of intense debate, mostly because of a looseness of terminology and the Freudian hangover. Freud related the loss of reproductive potential with mourning and melancholia. Indeed, it was common in our mothers' day for women in the

Change to be institutionalized. 'Nervous breakdown' it was called, because nobody associated their intense if temporary depression with the temporary breakdown of hormonal balance.

The concept of 'involutional melancholia' has been abandoned in recent years. The striking aspect of more recent psychoanalytic studies and psychiatric textbooks is their cavalier lack of almost any comment on the subject of the Change. Standard gynaecological textbooks still run through a laundry list of negative mental health symptoms said to be associated with the Change, but without tracking the positive changes in mental outlook as women emerge from the transition.

It is the women in their *mid-to-late forties* who show a peak in minor mental symptoms, in the five years immediately prior to the end of their cycles. Something changes profoundly, then, between the years of entry to this passage and the completion of it, when the hallmark is a euphoric burst of new energy. Yet the conviction persists in Western culture that the menopause precipitates a marked deterioration in mental health. And cultural attitudes swing tremendous weight in influencing how a woman copes at this time of life.

Seeking to correct this oversight, Dr C. B. Ballinger, an eminent Scottish psychiatrist, academic researcher and consultant at Royal Dundee Liff Hospital, found in a review of recent British and Dutch population surveys that 'complaints of "mental imbalance", fatigue, depression and irritability were most common in women who were still menstruating and reached a peak ... in women reporting irregular menstrual periods who could be considered immediately premenopausal.' Ballinger's own study confirmed that it was the women aged forty-five to forty-nine years *and still menstruating* who had the highest levels of negative mental effects. But she then followed up and found from population surveys that 'women in the postmenopausal years show less evidence of psychiatric disturbance than younger women'. Her conclusions are consistent with those reached by several other researchers using very different survey techniques.

The much-publicized Massachusetts Women's Health Study

reported in a 1986 Harvard Medical School publication that 'depression in middle-aged women is associated mainly with events and circumstances unrelated to the hormonal changes that occur at menopause'. Epidemiologist Sonja McKinlay, co-author of the study with her husband John, insisted in an interview: 'Most women just go straight through menopause, no problem. None, nor with irritability.'

Try out that line on a room full of menopausal-aged women and one is guaranteed a laugh. The McKinlays' conclusion – that depression at this stage is associated *only* with external 'social circumstances' – was suspect, since it was a paper-and-pencil questionnaire and no measurements had been taken of the actual hormone levels in peri- and postmenopausal women.

Of the many stories I had been told by women themselves, a typical description of menopausal malaise came from Nora. A former tavern owner, she was remarried as she started her forties and happily moved to the country. She had never been depressed before. At forty-six, when she began skipping periods, a fog of indeterminate sadness came over her from out of left field.

'I'd go out and walk for five miles every morning on a country road, sun shining, birds singing – and tears would start running down my cheeks. Why? I kept looking at my life – was there anything to validate this depression?' she recalled asking. 'Nothing. I was normally very up. My doctor told me I was too young for menopause. Then I remembered times in adolescence when I'd come home from school, go into my room, sit down on my bed and cry. That's when I knew. Whatever these doctors say, it's my hormones.' Her malaise, although frightening at the time, lifted within several months.

It is true that *clinical* depression subsides in women over fifty. And irritability and depression in middle-aged women do have many other sources. But mood changes are so commonly mentioned by women in the perimenopause phase, why should women be told there is no hormonal basis for feeling depressed?

'That's looking at major depression as a disease,' stresses Dr Howard Fillit, a gerontologist at Mount Sinai Hospital. 'A woman comes into a doctor's office at age fifty-one with the menopause and says, "Doctor, I can't function very well in the office. I think I have memory loss, I can't pay attention to my work and I feel really depressed." If the doctor reads the literature he knows that there's no major association of depression with the menopause, so he says, "C'mon, you're crazy." If the doctor was aware that these complaints and symptoms are real, although they may not qualify as a disease, this problem could be dealt with in a constructive manner.' Up to 80 percent of menopausal women in self-report studies describe feeling nervousness and irritability.

In fact, oestrogen does improve mood and the sense of psychological wellbeing even in well-adjusted women who have no distressing menopausal symptoms, according to a new study done by Dr Edward Ditkoff at the University of Southern California School of Medicine. Women in the random study who were given the standard dose of 0.625 mg of oestrogen a day showed a decided improvement in depression scores and were more optimistic and confident than those given a placebo. Neurobiologically, oestrogen has chemical effects on the brain that are similar to anti-depressants. The most experienced researchers say that when oestrogen levels in the blood are very low, a woman might start to feel a bit sad or blue, or notice irritability or mood swings, but not of a clinical magnitude.

That is the key distinction: women low in oestrogen often have feelings of malaise, as opposed to suffering from the *DSM-III* criteria of depression as disease (the criteria used in the McKinlays' Massachusetts study). Unless there are also underlying causes, the blues that may colour the years leading up to menopause are a temporary phenomenon.

Two areas of behaviour have been found by Dr Ballinger to be very widely influenced by menopause: sleep and sexual response.

Indeed, one of the most common sources of mood changes at this stage of life is broken sleep. Night sweats that awaken a woman several times, interrupting REM sleep night after night, can easily produce all the consequences of sleep deprivation. A major function of REM sleep is to allow important brain cells to rest and replenish their chemical stores, according to the latest dream research at Harvard Medical School. It also releases sleep-promoting transmitters and is crucial in regulating body temperature. So it should come as no surprise that a person awakened by temperature aberrations, and deprived of the REM sleep needed to reset the body's thermostat, is stuck in a vicious circle.

'These are real symptoms, don't think you're crazy,' Dr Robert Lindsay tells his patients. A good-humoured, Scottish-born endocrinologist, Lindsay was asked by New York State to set up a bone centre in conjunction with Columbia University. His clinic at the Helen Hayes Bone Center in West Haverstraw, New York is now booked almost a year in advance, because, he says, women are not getting reasonable answers to their questions about menopause elsewhere. 'The reason oestrogen works so well in curing menopausal depression is that it restores REM sleep,' he says. 'Once women can sleep better, they're fine. They don't need a psychiatrist or a divorce.'

To be sure, when Sonja McKinlay went back to do a five-year follow-up of the 2,570 middle-aged women in the Massachusetts study, she had to backtrack somewhat. Women who experienced a long perimenopausal period – more than a two-year transition – had a 'moderately increased, but transitory, risk of depression,' reports the 1992 paper. And this depression was prompted not by unfortunate social circumstances; it was due to menopausal symptoms. Still McKinlay holds out against the oestrogen deficiency hypothesis. 'If oestrogen deficiency caused depression, one would expect to see a continued high rate of depression beyond menopause, rather than a transitory peak.' But there may be a parallel here between puberty and perimenopause. In both instances, the effects on mood can be sharp but short-lived, as the body adjusts to a new hormonal milieu.

In my own earlier work, notably a study of wellbeing in

60,000 Americans undertaken by questionnaire with followup personal interviews and reported in my 1981 book, *Pathfinders*, life satisfaction among women was found to bottom out in the late forties. But it comes back strong in the early fifties, whereupon it goes from high to high. Most of the women who were between forty-six and fifty when surveyed showed clear evidence of passing through a danger zone. Coping strategies that had worked perfectly well for them in earlier stages did not seem to hold up against the volatile dips in optimism and blips of depression that characterized their late forties.

Facing the entryway of any new major passage in the life cycle is always far more daunting than actually moving through the transition. So many women in postmenopause have described to me, sometimes with bemused amazement, how vital and energetic and *focused* they feel. I was amused myself when I had a late lunch recently with a male friend in his mid-fifties. After walking thirty city blocks to the restaurant, I found my companion already halfway through his soup. 'I just couldn't wait,' he said. 'You're still going strong and you probably got up at six o' clock this morning.'

I was taken aback. 'How did you know?'

'Because women your age always seem to get up at six in the morning. You're more energetic than ever – just at the time we men are starting to wind down.' He was right about that switch, generally speaking, but such a comforting perspective is not real or believable for women until they themselves have actually come through the Change.

The passage of menopause is inextricably bound up with other common life events and cultural determinants. Harsh losses such as a parent's life-threatening illness or death are new and real around this time. The inescapable evidence of physical ageing and the cruel penalties of ageism also register. Women are brutally premature in disqualifying *themselves* as no longer attractive to men, simply because they are no longer young. And there is the artifact of generation. Few women in middle age today were prepared, professionally or emotionally, for the reality that being an earner becomes central to the self-esteem – and often the survival – of women in the middle years. The shift in body chemistry may be a casual matter compared with the faltering of one's former identity as the role of mother becomes distant and custodial, if not outright rejected. The menopausal identity crisis is exaggerated if one begins at the same time to lose social contact through divorce, retirement or widowhood.

Disengagement from the mothering role along with the end of fertility, however, turn out to be precursors to the beneficent change in body chemistry and mental outlook summed up in the term 'postmenopausal zest'.

So, despite the danger zone through which most women will pass in their late forties, a mobilization usually begins shortly after menopause, and a profound change in self-concept begins to register with rising exhilaration for many women as they move into their fifties. They often break the seal on repressed angers. They overcome the habits of trying to be perfect and of needing to make everyone love them. They may shed the terror of living without a man that trapped them in a dead or destructive marriage. Many women, during the decade of the mid-forties to the mid-fifties, find the sustained courage to extricate themselves from lives of desperate repetition.

The sense of wellbeing is more than happiness, the latter generally conveying relief from pent-up frustration or deprivation. Wellbeing registers deep in our unconscious, as a sustained background tone of equanimity – a calm, composed sense of all-rightness— that remains behind the more intense contrasts of daily events, including periods of unhappiness. On the life cycle graphs plotted from results of my 60,000 questionnaires, that sense of wellbeing gradually rises for women through the mid-fifties, reaching a high point around fifty-seven, when it takes off and soars. The issue of trying too hard to please is, for most, surmounted. Women begin at last to value *themselves*.

Several caveats must be added to these generalized statements on depression and menopause. Depression *is* correlated with surgical menopause. Most women feel relieved immediately after a hysterectomy. But a review of research by psychologist Ellen McGrath, editor of the American Psychological Association's 1990 task force report on *Women and Depression*, shows that women who have had hysterectomies are twice as likely to become depressed over time. The impact on sexual responsiveness and desire may be a major culprit. It is also likely that a woman who has suffered from phases of depression in the past will react in the same way during the transition of menopause.

The Massachusetts study confirms these observations. The two groups of women found most likely to become depressed are those who have experienced depression prior to menopause and women who have had hysterectomies. 'Depression *is* associated with surgical menopause, but it may be the cause rather than the consequence of the surgery since the group of women who undergo hysterectomies is atypical,' reports the study. Among those who were found on follow-up to have had the highest rates of depression, usually during perimenopause (apart from those with hysterectomies), were widowed, divorced and separated women with less than twelve years of education. Never-married women showed the lowest rates of depression. Married women fell between the two extremes.

Depression does become a widespread problem among older people in the UK. Relationships – just somebody to talk to – take on enormous importance. 'A lot of it is about networking,' says Terry Banks, supervisor of the Third Age Inquiry. 'When the obvious structures of family and work go, you've got to build your own network. In the States you may be ahead of us, generationally; networking is better established among older age groups. We still have a society, among the generation which is now in their fifties and sixties, where people were used to stable work and family structures. The idea that you have to construct networks for yourself, outside of defined groups, is actually quite frightening.'

Women who are used to having mood swings with PMS appear to be very sensitive to hormonal fluctuation, Dr Allen has observed in her practice. 'These women may be at risk for depression in the perimenopausal period, when hormonal fluctuations are unpredictable and most violent.' Again there is good news: such women experience great relief when they reach the postmenopausal period. They are released from the treacherous mood baths of their reproductive years and feel a consistency of calmness at last.

The acceleration of bone loss also begins during the perimenopausal phase, as do other changes in the long-term health status of the older woman. 'The problem is, nobody *feels* the bone they're losing until it's too late,' says Dr Lindsay. 'That is, osteoporosis is without symptoms until it becomes disease.'

We build all the bone we are going to make by the time we're thirty-five. 'Women really start to lose bone mass at forty,' says Richard Bockman, head of the endocrine department and co-director of the Osteoporosis Center at the Hospital for Special Surgery in Manhattan. 'Bone loss occurs rapidly even before the menopause, then accelerates during the menopause as hormones fall off, and eventually tapers off to a slower rate of loss about ten years after the onset of menopause.' Generally speaking, this timetable of bone loss occurs in all white women, according to the Osteoporosis Foundation in Washington, DC, though not necessarily for women of colour.

Similarly, silent changes in the blood vessels that nourish the heart begin taking place during perimenopause. Oestrogen makes a woman's blood vessels more elastic. Nature provides this relaxing hormone in abundance during the reproductive years because whenever a woman is pregnant her blood volume expands. If her blood vessels were as rigid as a man's, the increase in blood pressure would kill both mother and fetus in about the fifth month, according to Dr Estelle Ramey, professor emeritus and physiologist at Georgetown University.

'So all during your young years, whether you get pregnant or not, you walk around with more elastic blood vessels – until menopause,' says Dr Ramey. When a woman stops producing oestrogen, her 'good' cholesterol (HDL) level falls. 'Bad' (LDL) cholesterol levels start increasing during the transition *into* menopause, as confirmed by the National Institute of Health. Thus begins for women the narrowing of arteries that will gradually expose them to the cardiovascular disease from which oestrogen protected them during their fertile years.

In addition to noticing a lessening of lubrication in the vagina, many women also notice bladder problems or suffer the embarrassment of feeling a sudden urge to urinate before they can make it to the bathroom. This 'urge incontinence' is common, though little discussed, and may be associated with lack of oestrogen. Male urologists usually shun female patients with such chronic complaints. There may be no more than fifty female urologists in the United States. One of them, Dr Suzanne Frye in Manhattan, says there is a pill called Ditropan that can correct this bladder instability and change a menopausal woman's life.

'But I have cystic breasts, so I can't take hormones, right?' women would often ask in the group interviews. Cystic breasts are not uncommon at this stage. Dr Hiram Cody, one of the top breast surgeons at New York Hospital, explains, 'During the perimenopausal period breasts can become lumpier and more tender than before, due to surges of excess oestrogen. It subsides within a year after periods stop.'

Should women who are suffering the worst symptoms of menopause and accelerated health deficits be able to start hormone replacement therapy during perimenopause? The old dogma says no.

'We know now that there are good medical reasons for some women to begin hormone replacement therapy during the perimenopause years,' is how Dr Allen summarizes current practice. 'Acceleration of bone loss begins, risks for coronary artery disease start to increase, atrophy of breast and genital tissue starts. And so most doctors now believe that a woman who is bothered by menopausal symptoms, if she chooses HRT, should be treated before the cessation of her periods.'

As women wake up to perimenopausal problems and ask for treatment, American gynaecologists are increasingly recommending low-dose combination birth control pills to women in their forties. Oral contraceptives deal with the continuing risk of pregnancy even as they alleviate hot flushes and irregular or heavy bleeding.

'STRESS MENOPAUSE'

It used to be that a reliable guide to when you might expect menopause is when your mother experienced it. But the mothers of today's groundbreaking women knew nothing like the level of workplace stress and environmental toxins we live with today. Acute or prolonged and severe stress can reduce ovarian function and precipitate a temporary menopause at any time from the late thirties on. It may happen around the time of death of a close relative or other traumatic events. The phenomenon is similar to that experienced by a college student up against exams who misses a period.

An anaesthesiologist who deals with life and death every day, running an intensive care unit in a midwestern hospital, had her own life turned upside down in her fortieth year.

'I had a fire in my home that was rather devastating,' she recounts. Having out-stripped her own expectations, she was habituated to a high-performance life. 'Of course I said, oh, well, it was just a fire. I lived in a hotel for six months with two children to care for and continued working very hard – there was my team to run at the hospital – and I was determined that the fire would not have any impact on my life. It was just "pedal to the metal" and go right on.'

Noticing she was a little frantic, the anaesthesiologist began vigorously exercising an hour or two daily, in addition to her work and parenting responsibilities. She dropped down to a scrawny 105 pounds and couldn't sleep. 'I was anxious and depressed, though I didn't acknowledge it. Suddenly my periods, which have never been that regular, weren't around at all. And when I did sleep, I was waking up five or six times a night and throwing the covers off.' Her dentist husband said to her after a few weeks, 'Well, honey, I think you're in menopause.'

'What! I am only forty years old, of course I am not in menopause.' But the very next day, she did her blood test. 'My FSH and LH were off the wall and my oestrogen was very low,' she was chagrined to discover. 'It took me about five minutes to put an Estraderm patch on my behind [a means of delivering oestrogen through the skin], and within three days I felt my old self again,' continued the anaesthesiologist. After a couple of months, she stopped the exogenous oestrogen and her hormone levels remained normal. 'It seems I had a case of temporary menopause, due to much stress,' the physician diagnosed herself after the fact. It might also have been precipitated by the extreme weight loss, as found in young marathon runners with no body fat. 'In any case,' she says, 'I look upon that little visit of menopause as one of the greatest gifts that God has ever given me, because it made me quite sympathetic to older women.'

Everyone wants to be the person they were before. But your body is signalling that this is truly a change of life: you cannot put the same demands on it and expect it to be there for you whenever you have a period of high demand or unexpected stress. You cannot continue indefinitely being the same person as your younger self. To attempt it is the best way to precipitate depression.

Chemotherapy can also bring on a premature menopause. A head nurse at a major metropolitan hospital told me her personal story, which, sadly, is no longer unusual. 'I was diagnosed with breast cancer when I was thirty-seven and I had a mastectomy and a year of chemotherapy. It was the chemotherapy – the drug Cytoxin – that caused ovarian failure.'

The most unsettling aspect of this crisis period in the nurse's life was caused by her own – and her doctors' – ignorance about the impact of premature menopause. Known for her natural organizational skills and unflappable temperament, she had organized patient care in a high-demand environment for fifteen years. The untimely menopause caused her months of interrupted sleep and insomnia, along with mounting anxiety and feelings of depression.

'Suddenly, without any change of environment, my organization skills were compromised,' noticed the nurse. 'I was much slower. It was very troublesome.' Once the reason became clear, medication corrected the problems. Some women are lucky, however. Once the chemotherapy is over they do resume cycling naturally. But not all doctors are aware of these complications.

MENOPAUSE MUMS

Women having babies in their forties know they have departed from life cycle norms when they have to put on reading glasses to breast feed. 'I can't get him on the nipple without them!' squeals Sondra, the former sixties radical turned doting first-time mother at forty-two.

'I am the only self-avowed menopausal mother in my son's preschool,' was the amusing confession of Marcia Wallace, an American TV actress often seen on *The Bob Newhart Show* and *The Simpsons*. Marcia has cultivated the zany image of her celebrity with a red corkscrew-curled mop and loud colours and chandelier-sized earrings. But what struck me were the consequences of reversed life stages that her story represents. A late bloomer, Marcia devoted her young years to pursuing her career and postponed the personal commitments usually made by a woman in her twenties until she reached her forties. She married for the first time at forty-three.

'I figured, by then, all I had left was one egg on a walker,' Marcia quips. So she became an adoptive mother two years later. And a mere year after that – guess what? Marcia's new variant on women's life stages might be called The Compressed Life: marriage at forty-three, motherhood at forty-five, and menopause at forty-six.

A late first pregnancy often triggers an earlier menopause. An English woman who delivered her first child in her mid-forties found herself afterwards often drenched in sweat and gloomy. She told herself it must be post-partum depression (which is, indeed, rooted in the temporary depletion of oestrogen following childbirth). When the symptoms went on for two years, she began to wonder. But the last thing she would have done was to consult a doctor about menopause.

Her life became a maelstrom of role overload, marital strife, and eventually the failure of her own business and ensuing law suits. Always trying to do more, like so many women, she paid little attention to the needs of her body. When she began to have panic attacks and tearful outbursts over the least little setback, she sought out a Chinese medicine practitioner. The diagnosis: early menopause. She was stunned.

'I'm a young mother – how can you even think I'm an old lady in menopause!' she demanded.

The practitioner explained that the combined demands of a late pregnancy and stressful life events had taken a toll. Her metabolism had become very slow and her hormone level increasingly unbalanced. The depressed woman did not want to accept this reality. She insisted that her problems must be related to PMS, and that she'd always had them in milder form. She went on running on empty.

This is not an uncommon story today. The juxtaposition of a late pregnancy and early menopause can make the transition more psychologically painful, because it is so abrupt.

SEX AND THE
CHANGE-OF-LIFE LOVER

One subject women are least likely to bring up in connection with menopause is any change in sexual interest. The raging hormones of adolescence may suddenly become the *un*raging hormones of menopause. The British, in particular, 'are still frightfully po-faced about sex,' says MP Edwina Currie. 'They'll talk about almost anything, but if it's about *down there*, they won't talk about it.'

A high-profile American movie executive I know went through a major career move in her late forties, the sort of jump that inevitably kicks up gossip: *Was she fired?* One of her best friends warned her: 'You know, this could be a very bad mark on your career because people will say, "She's probably postmenopausal." You lose your value.'

'What are you saying!' the executive gasped in disbelief. 'A dried-up, over-the-hill, nasty old me? Do you really think that could be the perception out there?' From a distance, clad in a T-shirt, jeans and Top-Siders, the slim blond woman could still be mistaken for fourteen.

'Well, you *are* getting older,' warned the friend, probably projecting her own menopausal malaise.

'I was flushed with rage,' admits the executive. 'Because that meant I might be perceived as having no power.' She began brooding on her mother's experience. From family pictures she remembered that her mother had been 'cute' in her early fifties, but later in that decade, all at once, 'her whole face died'. So the executive had been spending more time on maintenance: getting her hair highlighted more frequently, going for collagen shots, doing lots of 'teeth things', dropping weight at a ritzy spa. Her first line of defence, she decided, would be to maintain her sex appeal and sexual energy.

'What's amazing is that at age fifty, I'm having the best sex I've ever had,' she told me confidently. Following a recent divorce, 'that part of me has suddenly come to life'. What does this have to do with menopause? Everything. Here is a woman who associates sexual potency with power, just like the men who have been her mentors and models at the top of corporate life.

'I made up my mind I'm not going to lose this part,' she said fervently. Menopause *will* be held at bay as long as she can keep up her sexual élan.

'Most women after the menopause, if they're reasonably healthy and happy, do not experience a diminution in sex drive,' says Dr Ramey, the senior physiologist at Georgetown University. 'But a very large number do – maybe 30 percent,' she estimates, adding that the figures are unreliable because doctors don't ask women about their sex drive. 'But since we're all living longer, this large number of women who face a diminished sex drive can be a very serious matter.'

It is particularly startling for women who have always been sensual to find even slight changes in intimate pleasures they have taken for granted. Gayle Sand is a case in point. A slinky, sexy-looking California woman with great black Diana Ross hair, she flew all the way to Manhattan to have her bone density measured at the Osteoporosis Center at the Hospital for Special Surgery – that's how jittery she was about this thing called menopause.

'I've always been a person that's looked much younger than I actually was. Even now I don't think I look forty-nine years old, do I?' She leaned back in the mean metal institutional chair, attempting a seductive nonchalance, and let the strap of her laminated white tank top drop off one deeply tanned shoulder at the two o'clock point, precisely where the swell of breast tissue started to come up off her ribs. Not an ounce of fat was discernible on her body, nor was there a line apparent in her face. But inside she was miserable.

'I've always taken really good care of myself . . . Look, it's like baby skin,' she said, holding out an arm glistening like a peeled peach. She was proud of having a DNA glow – all from a diet of boneless, skinless sardines she read about in the seventies in *Cosmopolitan*.

So what was she doing in an osteoporosis clinic, with all those brittle women suffering from low bone mass who have smoked and been slothful about exercise? Well, Sand's own mother had broken her pelvis. But we're not going to be like our mothers, are we? Sand belongs to the first generation of the new fifties woman. She has exercised almost every day of her life. 'So I figured I'd postpone all of this. It wouldn't even get to me. The first time I even thought about it was in an exercise class at Sportsclub-L.A. Dyan Cannon, Teri Garr, Magic Johnson, they all go there – it's the stars' gym. I see the tushies of everyone. There's hardly a woman there who has her own breasts. And you can be sure none of *them* ever had *menopause*.'

She was near the end of class, on the floor, grinding the old lower abs into the ground with leg lifts, when she started to perspire profusely. She thought, *What a great teacher!* 'But later in the afternoon I was in Gelsons – it's like one of the best supermarkets in L.A. – and I started to have that feeling again. Oh-oh, maybe it wasn't just the great instructor.' Dorian Gray time! *You're going to catch me being old.*

Sand was a dental hygienist: 'I cleaned the teeth of the stars.' She also had a new man in her life, a husband-to-be. She was in her psychiatrist's office when another hot flush hit, so she asked him about it. 'If I were you,' he said, 'I would never mention menopause to this man.' She followed the shrink's advice and hid her little secret from the man she married, which wasn't easy once she started having the night sweats.

Just beyond REM sleep – *bolt!*— she'd pop up like burnt toast. A minute later the sweating would start from every pore. Swiftly and silently she'd slip out from under the sheets and take a cold sponge bath, but sometimes her husband would awake and grumble, 'Hey, it's wet in here! Jesuschrise, whatsammatta with these *sheets*?'

'I'm just having a little anxiety,' she'd say, rubbing his head.

'But then around the same time your vagina starts to get dry. Also, I felt no desire.' Now she was talking about a flagging of libido as the oestrogen level drops and the tissues of the vaginal wall become thinner and drier. Imagine discussing *that* with your mate, said Sand. 'Unless you have a really decent guy, talking to him about menopause is like taking hemlock.'

She had learned from reading *Lear's* that yoga was the basis of Raquel Welch's regimen for reaching 'balance, calmness, and energy'. Of course, Raquel Welch, who at fifty looks like a low-fat-yogurt Lachaise, never mentions menopause. But Raquel does say the secret of remaining a sex symbol for ever is yoga. 'Change excites me. I am fifty years old. It's when the mind catches up with the body.' Along with a diet of Evian water, oat bran and protein-packed steamed salmon – that's all there is to it!

So Sand slid into bed as if she still belonged to a world of perfectly matched D-cup mango breasts and record arousal times, convinced that all she needed to do to enter the state of fifty-year-old erotica – the state of Raquel-mindedness – was 'the mere act of holding a position for a count of thirty or forty seconds'. She was thinking, 'I'll be a menopause centrefold. I have this glistening body, right? At the peak of a hot flush – You want a hot woman? *This* is a hot woman.' Her new husband manoeuvred her into position. And then, *it hurt.*

'It's hard to decide which came first, not wanting to have sex, or not wanting it because it hurt,' said Sand.

Finally, she sat her husband down and told him the facts of life. 'I'm going through my Change of Life.' Blank look. 'I'm going through menopause.' Her husband gave her a new name: my Change-of-Life Beauty Queen. She winced – it was a kiss with a kick.

'We find there's a definite major change in sexual response from premenopause to perimenopause,' concludes Professor Phyllis Mansfield from her past studies. 'The lessening of sexual desire is related to vaginal dryness, which suggests both hormonal and psychological factors.'

'Hormones primarily regulate sexual desire in human females,' points out Dr Kim Wallen, the primates researcher at Emory University. 'Among monkeys, what we could call middle-aged females are the most socially savvy and attractive to males, and sex is primarily initiated by the female.' When the researcher removed a half of the oestrogen they produce, some of the female monkeys continued to be sexually active, but when he removed all the oestrogen, they lost all interest in sex.

Virtually the same phenomenon has been demonstrated at McGill University in studies of women aged thirty to fifty whose ovaries had been surgically removed. Whether or not they took oestrogen orally after surgery, they were less interested, less aroused, and had fewer fantasies about sex. But while clinicians collect plenty of data on the frequency of intercourse, they seldom look at the key variable for females: sexual desire.

'There is an overall tendency among doctors to discount women's emotional needs,' observes Dr Wallen. 'They will spend a lot of time seeing if there's vaginal atrophy, but they won't spend any time asking about sexual interest or enjoyment.' This issue is still not seen as an appropriate part of a menopause workup. Yet a single woman without a regular sexual partner faces a different menopause than the married woman, since the former must be motivated if she is to find a mate.

In general, it can be said that women who enjoyed a lively sex life when they were younger are likely to go on enjoying – or missing – sex after menopause. Some psychoanalysts, like Graciella Abelin, a member of the International Psychoanalytic Association, hear a common confession from their female patients over fifty: *I've never been as aware of my sexual urges in my whole life.* 'Women are ashamed of this,' says Dr Abelin. 'The myth of ageing has conditioned them to believe that their sexuality should be going down the drain. They often feel that they are the exception, and they are embarrassed about being so sexual.' As their mates' potency declines, or they become widowed or divorced, some women over fifty seen by psychiatrists are turning to homosexual relationships with other women, when they had never considered that before. 'The female mates are more loving, and more accepting of the physical changes,' says Dr Abelin.

At the other end of the spectrum, postmenopausal women who come into the McGill University menopause clinic in Montreal, Canada, often say, 'The kids are gone, my husband and I like each other, we do lots more things together now. But I find I'm simply not interested in sex. Maybe I don't really love him.' Certain women notice the falloff in desire quite suddenly, says Dr Sherwin. 'When I can date it to the onset of menopause or several years thereafter, or to surgical menopause, in women who didn't have that complaint before, we suspect what they are missing is testosterone.'

Scientific measurements have established that testosterone level goes down by about one third in the average postmenopausal woman who still has her ovaries. If her ovaries are removed, the fall is twice as great. The figures come from an acknowledged expert in hormone measurement, Dr Howard Judd, Ob-Gyn professor at University of California, Los Angeles.

'Every woman has been told, "Don't worry, your adrenals take over," but the point is, the adrenals don't take over,' insists Dr Lila Nachtigall, associate director of the Women's Wellness Division at New York University medical school. The adrenal glands make about two thirds of the testosterone circulating in the body of young women. But from the age of thirty on, a woman's adrenal glands slow down. Preliminary studies by Dr Nachtigall show that after the ovaries are removed or shut down in postmenopause, the adrenal glands produce very little testosterone. What they do make is mostly in fat tissue in the body. 'So if the woman is thin, she also has less testosterone,' notes Dr Sherwin.

In some proportion of women the ovaries go on overtime – producing more testosterone even than during their reproductive life. These are the women who notice increased sex drive, and may see some hair appearing on their upper lip or chin. A woman who wonders about her testosterone level can have it measured from a blood sample; good norms exist.

Fay Weldon, the novelist known internationally for her wickedly wry chronicles of the battle between the sexes, observes in her recent novel, *Life Force,* '... when oestrogen levels sink in a woman, it is safe for society to give her hormone-replacement therapy, which keeps a female female, soft, sweet, and smiling, but antisocial to give the ageing man testosterone injections, for if you do he runs round raping women and hitting other men on the head. What a bummer!' In the novel four women of a certain age are revisited by the same old lover, Leslie of the Magnificent Dong, who is sixty years old but still intent upon using his vital ten inches to revive infidelities of the past. '... leaping, unstoppable, like electricity, from this one to that one, burning us up, making us old,' as one of his menopausal targets describes the experience. But testosterone for women? The intriguing possibilities hadn't yet occurred to Weldon. One can't wait to see what her imagination might do with that new wrinkle.

I visited Weldon in the leafy Kentish Town section of London. A great blond Valkyrie of a woman, feet planted firmly in the earth of her tiny townhouse garden, she was waiting outside to welcome me. We threaded our way through her sun-splashed work room, past a grown son slumped in a beanbag sofa on the phone, and into a small conservatory. All around were bunches of beautiful, blowsy late-summer roses, their petals splayed wide open, a rather apt simile for the attractive Earth Mother who sat before me.

In her mid-fifties, Weldon still sees sex as a necessary indulgence that both men and women need to survive. 'I suppose, by and large, men have more opportunity to be sexually active as they grow older,' she told me, 'but I think women remain more sexually alive.'

There is an important and poignant exception to this view, and Weldon herself would agree with it. It's what Germaine Greer is trying to get at when she talks about having rejected hormone replacement: 'When I used it myself, I didn't like that feeling of going back into the cycle,' she said in an interview on CNN. She had already been postmenopausal for a while, and having 'glimpsed another place' beyond sexual desire, she 'wanted to get back there'.

Greer claims that women over fifty who lose interest in sex are 'lucky'. Her belief, expounded to an amazed interviewer on CNN, is that 'you can live with no sex, but bad sex will make you crazy'. Sonya Friedman, the glamorous, happily married host of *Sonya Live*, took strong exception to Greer's view: 'Whether it's a good relationship or no relationship, I think a lot of women would like to feel that if they want sex, their body would be able to enjoy it comfortably.' But Greer seems to define her own superiority by dismissing middle-aged men, en masse, as fat smelly beasts whose sexual performance is grossly inferior to that of younger men. 'The thing they can't bear is that we don't need them,' she burst forth bitterly in another interview. 'Our indifference kills them. We don't need them!'

When one no longer feels competitive or graceful in the guise of sexual huntress, one might well take the attitude, 'Good riddance, who needs them?' The argument against hormone replacement then comes from an entirely new orientation: life without sex can be more peaceful and allow one to get more done. And, in truth, it may make some women happier than continuing along in the same state of emotional frenzy – open to humiliation, rejection, anxiety, and misery as well as to the pleasures of sex. The woman's underlying fear here is that after a certain age, her face can't be saved, her body is going, and she can't find a man. If one then takes the position that all men are beasts or sexually inferior, there is no need to admit that one doesn't really enjoy sex.

This may explain in part why some women start replacing their hormones, and then stop. While they were not circulating much of their own hormones, desire may have slowly ebbed. One doesn't really notice. But if it's restimulated by taking hormones, one realizes that there is always another level of sexual tension that runs along underneath, rendering one vulnerable to expectation and disappointment. Once it's back, and she is an older woman, her options are to satisfy it or to sustain an inconsolable longing. Throwing out the pills or patches, then, may have less to do with sore breasts or feeling puffy than the need to take herself out of play. Otherwise, she opens herself to hurt again. It's not easy to put one's finger on it, because the vulnerability is not just to sexual longing. It is opening oneself again to the possibility of being in love.

'Do I have to accept this?' is a question increasingly being asked by dynamic women in their fifties who are at the peak of their careers but alarmed to find their sexual pilot light abruptly lowered. Treatment with very small amounts of testosterone – always combined with oestrogen – is beginning to be popular. Dr Sherwin has had women on this combination of drugs, by injection, for up to twenty years, with good results. She cautions, however, that with a full dose of testosterone about 20 percent developed some facial hair. When she cut the dose in half, to 75 mg of testosterone once a month, less than 5 percent of women had any side effects. When given by injection, testosterone had no effect on HDL and LDL cholesterol levels.

Dr John Moran, a veteran Harley Street gynaecologist who has treated thousands of menopausal women over the past fifteen years, recommends a very weak testosterone called ProViron. With one half to one tablet per day – much less than the dosage recommended by the standard medical handbook – there seem to be no masculinizing side effects, but there is a subtle return of sexual vitality.

'For those postmenopausal women who find themselves having difficulty with arousal and reaching orgasm, a small amount of testosterone can make a big difference,' confirms Dr Ramey.

When I checked back with Gayle Sand, she had been told by a female doctor about topical oestrogen, a very low dose of Premarin used vaginally as a medication to maintain lubrication and keep tissue from thinning in the vaginal walls. 'The effects were great,' she exclaimed. 'I have a normal sex life again.' But she had also started a campaign to end the taboo. She'll speak up in an elevator: 'Is it warm in here, or am I having a hot flush?' When the occupants gasp, giggle, then cluck, 'You, you're too young for that,' Sand sings back, 'No, I'm not. I'm menopausal.'

Over-the-counter preparations can restore moisture to the tissues of the vagina *without* the use of hormones. Gloria Bachmann, Professor and Chief of Obstetrics and Gynaecology at the University of Medicine and Dentistry of New Jersey, along with Morris Notelovitz of the Women's Medical Center in Gainesville, Florida, conducted a one-year study demonstrating that Replens significantly increased vaginal health and quality of life in women suffering from vaginal dryness. The product works best when used on a continuous basis, rather than just prior to intercourse.

The UK counterpart, VagiFem, *does* contain oestrogen – but only a minute amount, 25 mcg. It is a particularly welcome solution for a woman who has had breast cancer and does not dare add more oestrogen to her system. The oestrogen in VagiFem does absorb into the blood during the first few weeks of application, but once the vagina becomes stronger, oestrogen absorption drops off. VagiFem remains only in the vagina and does not affect FSH levels.

'By and large, the women who have a problem with sexuality in middle life are old married women, like me,' believes Janine O'Leary Cobb, editor of *A Friend Indeed*, the Canadian menopause newsletter. (Address: P.O. Box 1710, Champlain, NY 12919–1710) 'Many of us feel we had great sex when we were younger, and we don't mind if we have less now.' But Cobb gets letters from women of fifty and fifty-two who have taken new, younger lovers. 'They're hot to trot and having a lovely time; sex was never so good.'

Thus is born a new Old Wives' Tale, in which women pass the word about the tonic effect of a Change-of-Life Lover. The head of a department at a prestigious university was in her mid-forties when she first heard about it from a woman in her mid-fifties. The older woman told her to look forward to menopause: pregnancy worries went out the window, and she'd had an affair of *grande passion* at that time – starting at forty-nine.

'I was stunned,' recalls the younger woman. She is petite and had always prided herself on being taken for younger than she was, but the habit of marriage to a man she had known for several decades had made a buried treasure of her erotic self. Then, suddenly, she found herself swept up in an affair. When? she smacks her forehead with the insight: 'It's only now I recognize *I* was the same age! Maybe I thought, *Forty-nine – last chance.*'

Gloria Steinem, known not only as the inspiration of the American feminist movement but as one of the most sexually animated women of her time, was delightfully frank when I asked her what a fulfilling sex life means to her now, having passed fifty.

'I am about to say a series of things that if I had heard them ten years ago, I wouldn't have believed them,' she laughed. 'All the readers of this should brace themselves – just have faith that it may be true for them too.' She laughed again. 'Sex and sensuality – going to bed for two entire days and sending out for Chinese food – was such an important part of my life, and it just isn't any more. It's still there, but it's less important. I don't know how much of it is hormonal and how much is outgrowing it.'

Her still-unlined face seemed more relaxed. She lay back against her sofa cushions, this peripatetic woman who never in the last eighteen years spent more than a few days at a time in her own apartment, and she looked, at last, at home. 'It doesn't really matter whether sex goes or doesn't go,' she summed up. 'What matters is that the older woman can choose whether it goes or not.'

Carmen Callil, the high-powered London publisher, chuckles when she thinks back on the 'revolting promiscuity' that she and her generation of the feminist vanguard engaged in during the sixties and seventies. 'I was obsessed with sex then,' she admits. 'But when you're younger, sex is about other things, too – adventure, boldness, identity.' Like Steinem, she never married. 'There's no doubt about it, I'm not as interested in sex as I used to be.' Sex has taken a place in her postmenopausal life comparable to television. Nice, but if she has something better to do, not now.

Germaine Greer, who states as baldly as any male sexist, 'I have always been principally interested in men for sex,' seems enraged because men are no longer interested in middle-aged women principally for sex. In championing the embrace of 'manlessness', Greer claims that half the women of menopausal age will be without a man in their bed anyway. This is a greatly exaggerated estimate. In the US March 1990 National Census, the percentage of forty-five to fifty-four-year-old women who were single, widowed, divorced, or married with a spouse absent totalled one quarter of their age group. The number of women in Great Britain between the ages of fifty to fifty-four who are single, widowed, or divorced totals 20.5 %, according to 1991 figures from the Office of Population Censuses and Surveys.

Happily married women or those who continue to enjoy having men in their lives cannot buy into Greer's militant celibacy, if they even believe she is serious. Newswoman Eve Pollard says, 'For those of us who are trying to juggle nine lives, including a long-term relationship with a man, the idea that because you stop menstruating, you should pack it all in, is nonsensical. I would be the first one to say, if you're not terribly happy with this boring man, and don't want to wash his socks, why wait till you have the menopause? Get out before. Who knows who you might meet?'

In sum, it may be vague melancholy, stimulated by the sexual aliveness revived by being on hormones, from which the physical symptoms are the excuse to withdraw. The very possibility of being open again to hurt causes so many women, discarded or ignored by men, to say, 'Why bother?' But in not bothering to revive their sexual desire, they may ignore caring for their bodies and mental wellbeing.

EDUCATING
YOUR MAN
ᴅᴠ

Most men go all twitchy when mention is made of anything to do with female reproductive organs or processes. They don't want to hear about your visit to the gynaecologist, and they'll do *anything* to get out of making a run to the shop to pick up tampons. There seems to be a hangover from primitive thinking that presupposes a woman is unclean when she is in cycle. And if she has 'female troubles', the last person she can count on for a supportive ear may be her man. Those deep inner spaces are supposed to be only for pleasuring; they are not meant to have clinical names or flesh and blood mal-functions.

Patriarchal and primitive societies have done their part in prescribing the menstrual taboo. Just as they have fostered a division of women into two dimensions – good little ovulating wife who is the passive receptacle, and the scarlet woman or witch, who is active, sexually dynamic, and terrifying – men in traditional cultures have isolated the menstruating woman as 'unclean', 'polluting', and 'dangerous'. One would logically think that the woman who is finished with the fearsome busi-ness of monthly bleeding would become better accepted, and in some traditional subcultures she is. But there is a new, subjective fear, and not just in primitive societies.

Middle-aged men, as they themselves begin to slow down, have a good deal of fear and envy of the physical, mental, sexual, and spiritual energies of fully evolved women – women who are beyond being objects defined by the male gaze and now fully conscious keepers of their own bodies. That fear is projected back on to women, causing us to wonder if we really are over the hill when we no longer have value primarily as erotic objects and reliable breeders.

In fact, married men are more apprehensive about the effects of menopause on their life satisfaction than women themselves. In a 1991 gallup poll commissioned by Ciba-Geigy, makers of the Estraderm patch, one in four of the seven hundred women aged forty to sixty expressed concern about menopause, but two thirds of the middle-aged husbands were bothered about it. Only a third of the women were satisfied with their husband's knowledge about the Change of Life, and with good reason. Two thirds of the husbands of premenopausal women expressed fears that their sex lives would be compromised by having a wife in menopause. A majority of the men married to women in the transition focused on the emotional impact on their wives, saying they manifested anxiety, irritability, and mood swings. Fewer than half the men took any notice of physical problems that underlie these emotional reactions, despite the fact that the overwhelming majority of the women in menopause reported struggling with hot flushes, night sweats and difficulty sleeping.

A gynaecological nurse at New York Hospital is struck by how men shun their wives when they come into the hospital for a hysterectomy. 'The absence of the husband when it's an issue of female sex organs is so common', says Tanya Resilard. 'And if they do come to visit, they seem afraid to go to the bedside. They want to be totally separate.'

'My husband was incredibly supportive when I had breast cancer, but he really doesn't want to acknowledge I'm in menopause,' I was told by a gutsy entertainer. Her spouse is a few years younger than she. When she tries to talk to him about having problems with concentration, he ascribes it to something else – it's stress or money problems or maybe flu – anything but the Change of Life. 'He is in major denial about it – why?'

If you are getting older, so is your man. You may represent the mirror of his own ageing. Breast cancer a husband can't catch. But ageing is sex neutral. Another woman who felt constrained about admitting to her husband she was struggling with menopause finally realized why. She was the second wife and represented to the husband his own renaissance. 'He once told me, "I don't ever want to think of you as middle-aged".'

In fact, there is much to recommend a woman nearing the end of her reproductive stage. With the passing of pregnancy fears, her lustier fantasies can be played out with a refreshing lack of inhibitions. Best of all – and she must boast about this – she is soon to be free of the 'blue meanies' that come with monthly cycles. The Gallup poll findings support this good news: living through menopause puts far less strain on marriages than the apprehensions would suggest. A nearly identical majority of the husbands and wives polled – 70 percent – acknowledged that in fact the women's interest in sex had not decreased during or after menopause. And two out of five of the women presently in the transition or just past it say that their relationship with their husbands has improved since menopause, while the majority of women reported the quality of their marriages has remained the same.

If there are physical problems or discomforts, they do need an honest airing. The consequences of not being honest with your man about what's going on can magnify the psychological burden and become devastating. Two middle-aged men came to hear a talk I gave on menopause at a health resort. I was delighted to see them in the audience but curious as to why they would join a group of fifty women. Each of them came to me in his own time to unburden himself. 'I had no idea what women go through in these years,' said the trial lawyer, who later stretched beside me after a hike. 'My wife may be silently suffering.' He sounded seriously concerned, even abashed. 'I'm going to talk to her about menopause as soon as I get home.'

A New York lawyer caught up with me as we were boarding the plane and seemed to need to talk. 'I think men need to be educated about menopause even more than women,' he said.

'Your wife is a lucky woman,' I quipped. My remark set off a shudder of pain in his face, though he said nothing further. Later, over coffee, he told me that his wife had exhibited many of the symptoms I had described. 'The sweating at night, insomnia, problems with concentrating. Her moods were up and down, and then mostly down. I had no idea what it was.'

Further conversation revealed that his wife had lost her job as a teacher in the recession. Their son had moved out to his own apartment. And she had brought her mother up from Florida to care more attentively for her, but the frail woman had liver cancer and soon died. All in all, a rather typical portrait of the stresses of social as well as physical change many women experience during the menopausal years.

'I guess I just didn't stop to think how much these losses meant to her. And on top of it, the drain of menopause,' he said, flooded with guilt. I tried to comfort him and suggest new approaches for the future. It was too late. One day, four months before, his wife had driven him to their suburban train station for his commute to the city. She knew he had a late dinner with the senior partner that night. When he came home, he noticed the window of the garage door milky. He found his wife entombed in the car.

The
Menopause
Gateway

Some women have genetic good fortune. Even after entering menopause, they continue to make enough female hormone precursors in their adrenal glands, and to make enough oestrogen from these precursors in their fat deposits, so that they do not experience any symptoms, or at most, only temporary hot flushes. This pause is a marker event in their lives, but it does not take on the physical or psychological freight of a major event.

'They are thrilled not to have to deal with the menstrual cycle any more and some of them seem to maintain their bone levels very well,' observes Theresa Galsworthy, the nurse clinician who directs the Osteoporosis Center at the Hospital for Special Surgery in New York. Broad-scale figures on the proportion of women who fall into this fortunate group are probably impossible to come by, but activity at the Osteoporosis Center offers a clue. 'During the course of the week, about fifteen patients come to me to have their bone density measured because they're fairly newly postmenopausal. Maybe two or three of the fifteen have absolutely no symptoms,' says Galsworthy. These women are usually on the older side of the norm when they experience the Change, fifty-one or fifty-two.

Women who deal with menopause by denying it entirely become easy to pick out. They are the ones you see lunching on a lettuce leaf and glass of seltzer, their hair colour slightly lurid, their time more and more taken up with becoming skilful makeup artists or searching for the right cosmetic surgeon. The results may be admirable, and mask the years, but sooner or later time and nature will catch up with us all.

Strenuous dieting at this age, for instance, is the worst way to preserve one's long-term health and grace. Oestrogen is stored in the body's fat cells. Some researchers differentiate between the Thin Woman's Menopause and the Plump Woman's Menopause, the latter usually being far less symptomatic. 'In populations where women don't get carried away with wearing a size 6 dress when they're fifty-five, and they still do regular exercise and they're not smoking, bone fractures are not much of a problem,' says Dr Elizabeth Barrett-Connor, a top epidemiologist at the University of California, San Diego.

At the opposite extreme are women who allow themselves to become 'victims' of menopause, using this time of life as an excuse to become inactive, go to fat, beg off sex, and sulk, often leading them to depression and the door of menopause clinics. These are the middle-aged women who perpetuate the stereotype of the menopausal woman as synonymous with 'mean old bitch'.

The professional women I have studied are accustomed to considerable control over their environment and they have worked hard to achieve it. They pride themselves on being fiercely organized and prepared for just about any crisis. These mid-forties dynamos can fax a dinner menu to a caterer, sell a stock, talk supportively to a spouse over a portable phone without missing a step, and remember to take their aerobics shoes to the office along with their satin slingbacks so they'll be able to exercise before appearing glamorous at the AIDS benefit – all this on the way to do cancer surgery. But they cannot control when they break out in a hot flush or when they bleed.

The meanest loss of menopause, for them, is the sudden loss of control. Among high-performing professionals, puzzlement often develops into panic followed by outrage. That was the

route travelled by Meredith, a mother of two and model business leader in her middle-American community, who had
stopped counting birthdays at thirty-eight. That was the year
she went into business and consciously knew she looked terrific and felt the same way.

She started having mysterious migraines at forty-two. They
grew more frequent. Over the next ten years she traipsed
around to one gynaecologist after another, all of whom posited
psychological causes: i.e., 'Type A's are often migrainous.' At
age fifty Meredith was the one to insist upon a blood test that
would measure her hormones. She had zero oestrogen and
zero progesterone. Now completely frustrated, she saw a TV
commercial for a menopause clinic in Cleveland, Ohio. She
flew there to have a bone densitometer test, which revealed
she had 10 percent less bone mass than the norm for women
her age. Not one doctor up to then had mentioned her bones
in connection with menopause or brought up the risk of osteoporosis.

'I feel like I dropped a percentage point of bone mass in
each one of those doctors' offices,' Meredith says ruefully. She
also wonders, with good reason, if the migraines were the
result of oestrogen depletion over the past ten years.

I recognized her immediately when we first met. It was the
walk, perhaps. Her long legs took the sidewalk one full paving
stone at a time, high heels notwithstanding. She was good-
looking, still blond and pink-complexioned, the parentheses at
either side of her mouth lending animation to her face. Her
friends had described her as 'dynamic, tough, successful, and
doesn't take no for an answer'. Her real estate company will do
fifty-five million dollars of business this year and her mortgage
banking company will do eighty million.

'You'd think I could manage my period, right?' Meredith
wisecracked. Fifty – the number itself – held no menace for
her, she said, although it came out that the year Meredith
turned fifty, her mother died of breast cancer. It was her first
personal experience with death, immediately followed by the
onset of menopause. 'And something happened to me, I don't
know what, I became a little nutsy about flying in an airplane.

I began to feel a foreshortening of time.' Meredith said she was too busy to figure it out.

'I've been obsessed,' she says. 'Menopause is the only thing that's made me feel I had an age. Because I can't get rid of it. I hate it, big time.'

During a group interview, Meredith held up the computerized cost-benefit chart she had designed to analyse whether or not to take hormone replacement therapy. The impressive-looking graph was all the more infuriating to her because there was no bottom line. 'So what do I go for? Cancer, osteoporosis, or heart disease?'

For her, menopause represents her lack of control over mortality. Most of us don't have to face up to mortality until our mothers die. The loss of that unconditional love leaves no cushion between ourselves and the outrages of life, no grip against a suddenly perceived slippage on 'the downward path' toward one's own inevitable 'dusty death'. Control becomes magnified in importance. In reaction, Meredith developed her new phobia about airplanes, where as a passenger she could exercise no control. Still, she had pushed away any conscious recognition of her own ageing, until the physical insults of menopause finally made it impossible to remain, even in her own mind, thirty-eight.

Now, faced with making a medical decision about her own life that involves the breast cancer issue, with the loss of her mother not yet mourned, Meredith is in a constant state of conflict. She longs to escape from her own success: 'Being a mentor is a burden. I feel like I don't live anything new.' She resents her husband's assumption that he will take early retirement. 'What about me?' I feel like saying. 'When can I retire?' She is unconsciously afraid that she will follow her mother before she has had time to live fully. All these fears and frustrations have been focused on the secondary issue of menopause. And they come out as anger.

To make matters more frustrating, the cost-benefit analysis on how to treat menopause resists adding up to any clear, rational, risk-free answer. Why? Because we don't have enough data. And because everything has a price. A well-informed, affluent woman like Meredith might well decide, 'Well, hell, if I know hormones are going to protect my heart, my mind, and my bones, I guess I can monitor my breasts with mammography and my uterus with ultra-sound, and see how it goes.' Or, she may prefer to try to manage the whole process naturally.

PARTNERING YOURSELF THROUGH A NATURAL MENOPAUSE

Many women resist medicalizing a natural event such as the Change. Others, like Serafina Corsello, have little choice.

'I had a wonderful defence, called denial,' admits Dr Corsello, an elegant European woman who practises nutritional medicine at the Corsello Center on Manhattan's West Side. She was simply never going to have all those unseemly symptoms other women report, poor things. Blessed with high energy and an insatiable desire for learning beyond dogma, Corsello completed a medical internship and residency in New York. Throughout her thirties she juggled a classical medical practice with being a single mother. But in her early forties she became disenchanted with mainstream medicine. The outcome of her midlife crisis was a commitment to educate herself in complementary medicine – vitamin therapy and other natural procedures – realizing that it meant she would have to study every day for the rest of her life.

'Will I be able to keep up this level of performance?' she worried as she plunged into self-education, taking on new financial burdens as well as committing to a second marriage. But at fifty she found she still had fantastic energy, having always been able to hit the pillow and sleep within two seconds.

'At fifty-two, all of a sudden I'd hit the pillow, and hit the pillow – at two in the morning I'd still be hitting the pillow. This was the first sign; it was devastating.'

It took Dr Corsello no time to get an oestrogen patch and congratulate herself on re-regulating her sleep. She was herself again for the next two years. 'One day I woke up and felt an ominous mass in my breast.' Suddenly aware of the history of cancer in her family, she looked at her lovely little patch and progestin pills and said, '*Adieu, chérie.*'

She doctored herself with Chinese herbs, indulged in a massage once a week, and concentrated on creating a new aesthetic in her life. She surrounds herself with classical music – even in her office it is constantly in the background, soothing her. Since she loathes exercise but loves dancing, Dr Corsello built in her own unique daily stress-reducing activity. She shuts the bedroom door while she watches a tape of the MacNeil/Lehrer News Hour and throws herself into high-paced disco dancing, all by herself.

Today age fifty-eight, vivacious and utterly charming, Serafina Corsello has just signed a ten-year lease on her office in Manhattan – a powerful statement of her belief that 'I'm not only in my prime now, but I'm on my way up.' Like many professional women, she is operating under a different time line than her male peers. Her career development was delayed by single motherhood, and slowed slightly by menopause. 'I cannot stop at sixty, because I have hardly begun,' she says enthusiastically. But there is nothing stopping her now. She works every day, and on weekends she studies and writes. 'The constant intellectual stimulation allows my mind and body to remain attuned. I keep on improving,' she says.

The greatest reward of fifty-plus years of experience, she finds, is mental efficiency. She can actually sense her right and left brains, working in synchrony. And with this wide spectrum of intellectual capacity, she says, 'We can zoom in to get the whole picture.' She now expresses her ideas on health care *without fear* of offending the male medical establishment. She

no longer labours under the younger woman's apprehensions
– 'What if I'm not right?' or, 'Oh my god, will they be
offended?'

'Do you know how much energy this saves?' she says,
twinkling. 'I used to go into preambles – "you know" and "on
the other hand" – but I've cut fifty percent of that – it's freedom!' As she says now, 'If I'm not right, well, I'm not right.
This attitude allows you to shortcut all the tangents you had
to go through as a young woman – because, no longer being
a sexual object, you're no longer trying to *please* anybody. At
this point what is important to me is elegance. And elegance
has nothing to do with sex.' The greatest change she has
noticed is the aesthetic confidence she has developed as an
older woman.

Dr Corsello has explored most of the herbal preparations
popularly used to ease menopausal symptoms. She finds the
most effective to be dong quai, a Chinese herbal remedy. 'If
I'm under stress, bingo, I take thirty or forty little drops and
find miraculous relief.' She suggests a woman ask a Chinese
herbalist to make up a mixture to suppress hot flushes.

Dong quai, the Chinese herb, contains plant sterols that
have oestrogen-like effects. Plant oestrogens are one four-
hundredth as strong as the oestrogen from pregnant mare's
urine found in Premarin, estimates Janet Zand, a Chinese
medical practitioner in Los Angeles. Dong quai is available
in health food stores in tiny black beans. Siberian ginseng is
the herbal equivalent of testosterone and is helpful in opposing
fatigue and depressive symptoms. It, too, is available in health
food stores, or easily taken as Ginseng tea.

The theory in Chinese medicine is that energy in the
kidneys begins to decline for women around the age of forty-
nine, and so it was written in the ancient Chinese texts. Today,
a Chinese medicine practitioner would assess the individual
woman and make up a mixture of herbs to revitalize her kidney
function.

The Indian homeopathic tradition, as practised by the
world-renowned Shyam S. Singha, who has several clinics in
London and one in Suffolk, is to treat menopause entirely

through diet and homeopathic remedies. He finds the agnus castus herb particularly helpful in rebalancing oestrogen and progesterone levels. He also recommends dolomite, a mineral rich in magnesium and calcium; almonds, soaked overnight and peeled are also very rich in calcium. Some women report they obtain relief from hot flushes and sweats from acupuncture.

Vitamin E is commonly used to relieve hot flushes. Primrose oil is another longstanding remedy. It contains gamma-linoleic acid, which helps to mediate hormonal activity.

The best natural defence against osteoporosis is to keep the acidity of your blood in proper balance. If you don't, your body will, removing calcium from your bones to defend the pH balance in the blood. Blood acidity is caused, first and foremost, by chronic stress. Therefore, it is of the utmost importance for any woman over forty-five faced with high-stress professional or personal demands to commit herself to some restorative relaxation measure. It might be biofeedback, prayer, yoga, or routine meditation.

I find much wisdom in the ancient Hindu health system known as Ayurveda. The guiding principle is that any disorder can be prevented as long as balance is maintained, in the mind and spirit as well as in the body. Dr Deepak Chopra, one of the first medical doctors to introduce Ayurvedic theory and practice in the West, explains in his book, *Perfect Health*, 'The mind exerts the deepest influence on the body, and freedom from sickness depends upon contacting our own awareness, bringing it into balance, and then extending that balance to the body. This state of balanced awareness, more than any kind of physical immunity, creates a higher state of health.' From modern science we know that the hypothalamus, or 'the brain's brain', is responsible for balancing everything that goes on automatically in the body. Less than an ounce of grey matter in the forebrain must simultaneously balance the body's temperature, rate of metabolism, and sleep, along with its growth, hunger, thirst, blood chemistry, respiration, and many other functions. For optimum health to be maintained, coordination by the hypothalamus must be as precise as the movements of a conductor with a 150-piece orchestra.

During the perimenopause and early phase of menopause, even the brain's brain is often thrown off by the unpredictable changes in a woman's internal hormonal milieu. Try as it might, sending desperate signals to the pituitary gland to activate more oestrogen, the hypothalmic regulator is confused when the ovaries don't respond as they did before. It can't do its usual conducting job. Hence, the body is often out of balance. Good health is harder to maintain.

Many women will develop allergies for the first time during the menopausal transition. If the state of imbalance is allowed to become too extreme, and the immune system is weakened, the disease process sets in. Everyone recognizes the sensations that presage an oncoming cold or flu, even though they are vague. Similarly, a menopausal woman whose body is seriously out of balance will feel 'out of sorts', tired, cranky, and may complain of vague discomforts that are the body's premonition of disease.

Most doctors are baffled or impatient with such reports (if a woman even thinks her complaints serious enough to take to a doctor). Unless a woman takes herself seriously, and invests some time in learning about her vulnerabilities at this time of life, she may wind up with illness.

What can you do for yourself? The single most important aid to continued health through the menopausal transition is proper rest. When you feel that you are pushing yourself too hard, or racing, stop and rest if only for five minutes. Even better, learn how to meditate. The most restful rest, aside from a night's sleep, is the deep relaxation experienced during the state of meditation. According to Dr Chopra, the common symptoms of the 'worried well' in menopause – headache, insomnia, low-level anxiety or depression – benefit most from the act of meditation. One can emerge thoroughly settled and refreshed after only a few minutes of transcending.

It is not wise to drink alcohol or too much coffee while you are trying to rebalance your body. Moreover, to minimize loss of mineral from bone it is vital to keep the acidity level in your blood as low as possible. Smoking, alcohol, and coffee also raise acid levels in the blood. Even a nightly glass of wine can wreak havoc with a hormonal system already out of balance. Carbonated sodas and beef, both of which have a high phosphorus content, are particularly dangerous for post-menopausal women, advises Dr Corsello. She suggests a diet that emphasizes vegetables, complex carbohydrates, fibre, fish, and vegetable proteins such as tofu.

We know that Japanese women, who enjoy the fewest symptoms during menopause and the most robust health thereafter, eat a daily diet including tofu. Tofu is made from soya, and soy contains oestrogen. It behoves Western women to think about altering their diet.

No natural remedies can be guaranteed effective. Bear in mind that no pharmaceutical company stands to cash in on herbal remedies, since they are natural and can be sold over the counter. And since drug companies fund much of the medical research, it is not surprising that there is no serious money going into the study of Chinese medicine and its impact on menopause.

The pledge to have a 'natural menopause', while politically correct, presents some contradictions. Is it 'natural' to live for decades beyond fifty? And to want to feel in our seventies the way we do now?

This will be the first generation to get old routinely, and one way or another its women will have to provide some things that mother nature did not. None of the herbal remedies protect against bone loss. And no herbs or holistic inter-cessions will prevent changes in the sex organs. Oestrogen is what causes the vagina to moisten when aroused. As oes-trogen levels decline, the vaginal tissues become thinner and dryer. Gradually, over the decade of menopause, the vagina will shrink in both length and width. One female gynaecolo-gist drew me a picture of the normal oestrogenized vagina of a woman in her thirties. It looked about five inches long and the width of two middle fingers.

'In many women of sixty who have taken no oestrogen,

I can hardly insert my pinky,' said the gynaecologist. If a woman discontinues hormone replacement, the process of atrophy will start again. Doctors recommend that older women keep up an active sex life because that will keep the vaginal walls elastic. But the common reason that women don't 'use it' and eventually 'lose it' is because making love becomes naturally painful when the vagina shrinks in size. Oestrogen cream, as explained, and new over-the-counter preparations do counteract the discomfort.

THE HIDDEN
THIEVES

Active women often take pride in toughing it out: 'I was too busy to notice menopause – I just sailed right through it' is their refrain. They may not be fully aware of the hidden thieves of menopause: osteoporosis, cognitive changes, and heart disease. We must be aware of these dangers before any of us can make an intelligent decision about how best to manage our own menopause.

Start up a conversation with any group of women where the ratio of blond to grey has tipped well over the fifty-fifty standoff, and there will be one woman who proclaims righteously, 'Hormones, not me! I want to stay healthy.' Another will insist smugly, 'I love my oestrogen, I wouldn't give it up for anything!' And another will be totally ambivalent, able to be talked into either decision. Elizabeth Barrett-Connor, the University of California epidemiologist, observes that women break down into these three camps.

Most women have become phobic about breast cancer, with some good reason. Their fear, however, leaves them vulnerable to a greater threat. At each group interview I asked the participants to guess what they were most likely to die from. The answers always startled me. Nine out of ten women will say cancer, most of them specifying breast cancer. A few will throw in the possibilities of airline or car crashes. Almost no one mentions the number one killer of women over fifty.

Heart disease.

In fact, *a woman's chances of dying from heart disease are more than double that of dying from cancer of any kind.* Even as the rise in breast cancer among women continues apace – one in *nine* women are now diagnosed and one in four of those will die from breast cancer within five years – cardiovascular disease quietly kills off one in *two* women over the age of fifty.

THE CHEATING
HEART

Although the risk of heart attack does not increase abruptly at the moment a woman reaches natural menopause, the rate of heart disease does rise sharply over the course of the decade after a woman reaches her fifties. A clear picture of the 'cumulative, absolute risks' of the major causes of death for white women – between the ages of fifty and ninety-four – were spelled out in an editorial accompanying the Nurses' Health Study. There is a 31 percent absolute risk of dying of heart disease, a 2.8 percent risk of dying of breast cancer, a 2.8 percent risk of a hip fracture, and only a 0.7 percent risk of uterine cancer.

'Then why don't we read about women having heart attacks the way we do men?' someone will sensibly demand.

Perhaps because doctors pay less attention to women's symptoms of heart disease and treat them less aggressively than they do men. As a result, women often develop more advanced heart disease and are more likely to have a fatal heart attack than men. Two new studies involving tens of thousands of patients have recently shown irrefutable evidence of sex differences in the way heart conditions are treated. The unawareness of the general public simply reflects the prevailing attitude in the medical fraternity that heart disease is a man's disease.

'Women lag behind men in heart disease by about five to seven years,' says Dr Trudy Bush. 'It really starts hitting women in their late fifties and sixties.' By the age of sixty-seven they are just as likely to have a heart attack as their husbands, but more likely to die from it.

The most significant predictor of heart disease is the HDL level. 'Bad' cholesterol levels normally increase in women for some ten to fifteen years following the cessation of periods. Again, dangerous changes in cholesterol count or blood pressure do not announce themselves with obvious symptoms, not until there is a medical catastrophe. 'If your HDL level is low, and your LDL level is relatively higher – even if you're walking around with a total cholesterol count of two hundred – you're going to be in trouble,' says Dr Ramey. Oestrogen replacement therapy decreases LDL (bad) cholesterol levels by about 15 percent, and raises the HDL (good) cholesterol levels by the same amount.

Oestrogen has a direct effect on the wall of the blood vessels. 'Cholesterol uptake is the first change that occurs in the creation of the plaque that forms the basis for heart disease,' explains Dr Lindsay. 'Oestrogen appears to block that effect, resulting in open vessels and good blood flow.' That explains why oestrogen reduces heart disease.

The Nurses' Health Study, the first prospective study of women's health with a population of tens of thousands of women (almost exclusively white), has found striking results on the heart disease front. After ten years, forty-eight thousand of the subjects, who had no history of cancer or heart disease when the study began, were evaluated. 'Women who were taking oestrogen after menopause had just half as many heart attacks and cardiovascular deaths as women who never used oestrogen,' reported Meir Stampfer, who led the study. An evaluation by Dr Lee Goldman of Brigham and Women's Hospital in Boston concludes, 'The benefits of oestrogen outweigh the risks, substantially.'

EMBEZZLED BONE

The second major thief of menopause is osteoporosis.

Margie is very good at giving care to everyone else – her laundry-toting post-adolescent kids and the battered women she works with at the community centre in her college town. Still blond, though aware she is white at the roots, Margie will turn fifty this year. 'Oh, shit, my number's up,' was her reaction. Her doctor told her ten years ago she was a sitting duck for osteoporosis. Small-boned, she remembers her statuesque mother shrinking about seven inches to a mere five feet tall before she died. 'I already know I have bone thinning,' she admits.

Typically, she resists addressing the issue because that would mean goodbye to youth. 'I'll take hormones when I get there.'

'What's *there*?' her girlfriend challenged her.

'You know, old.'

Old is too old to start protecting bones. By the time anybody can *see* osteoporosis, it's too late to reverse it. As you'll recall, we begin to lose bone after the age of thirty-five; the normal rate of loss is about one percent a year. 'When you hit fifty, bone loss accelerates to about a percent and a half each year for about ten years,' says epidemiologist Trudy Bush, quoting the studies. 'Then it levels off again at one percent a year.'

Two factors determine a woman's risk of having significant

bone loss during this transition. First, her genetic background, and here nature turns the tables on our Western beauty ideal. 'I could look at a woman and bet her risks of osteoporosis: fair-skinned, very thin, a smoker, and an early menopause – and usually they'll be symptomatic,' says Dr Lewis Kuller of the University of Pittsburgh School of Public Health.

The second factor is: how strong are the bones a woman has built at her peak? About one third of American women of all ages are calcium-deficient. 'The preoccupation of teenage girls is with thin thighs, not good bone, so they get into the habit of drinking diet soda instead of milk,' laments Dr Barrett-Connor. But generational differences here are striking. The frail women who are now immobilized in nursing homes are a different breed from baby boomers who are out there bouncing from work to gym in their nitrogen-cushioned aerobic shoes, popping calcium and snacking on veggies. In Britain, women currently in their fifties and sixties are at particularly high risk because of deprivations in their diet as youngsters growing up during the Second World War.

Porous bones, which lead to increased risk of fractures, are a major public health problem. One third to one half of all post menopausal women – and nearly half of all people over age seventy-five – will be affected by this disease, maintains the National Osteoporosis Foundation in the US. Almost a third of women aged sixty-five and over will suffer spinal fractures. And of those who fall and fracture a hip, one in five will not survive a year (usually due to postsurgical complications).

Similarly daunting figures apply in the UK. Before a charitable trust appeared on the scene about five years ago to publicize it, 'osteoporosis' wasn't even on the map. Most doctors dismissed it as part of the normal process of ageing. Linda Edwards, deputy director of Britain's National Osteoporosis Society, gives a grim picture even today. Conservatively, she estimates that two million out of the eleven million postmenopausal women in Britain suffer from osteoporosis. Of that two million, only seventy-six thousand are given a prescription for their bone loss. Half of them have actually fractured a vertebra. But when they go to their GPs complaining of back pain, their fractured vertebrae are not recognized. And so, of those seventy-six thousand, 90 percent are being given only painkillers or calcium. 'In other words,' sums up Edwards, 'they are not getting any actual treatment at all.'

The National Osteoporosis Society has mounted a Herculean effort to raise awareness of osteoporosis through the media and to put it on the medical agenda as a reality with very serious health consequences for *young* women as well as old – 'because we consider the fifties as young,' adds Linda Edwards. She emphasizes a preventive approach: 'There are things you can do for yourself to *put bone in the bank.*'

Untreated, older women not only die from the consequences of osteoporosis, it often leaves them frail, susceptible to falls and broken bones, as well as to the little tortures of hairline fractures in the bones they use for walking and bending – and this by their sixties. Later, in their seventies, osteoporosis makes it painful merely to sit on hip bones pulverized almost into powder; it keeps many women homebound, later even chairbound, and is one of the primary reasons an independent woman will finally succumb to nursing home admission.

Taking calcium supplements *alone* cannot undo the damage done by the loss of oestrogen during the period of accelerated loss. And contrary to conventional wisdom, exercise *by itself* is also ineffective in preventing bone loss. These were the results of a study on prevention of postmenopausal osteoporosis reported in the *New England Journal of Medicine* (24 October, 1991). Two regimens were found to be effective. An exercise programme *plus* calcium supplements slowed or stopped bone loss. The best results were obtained when oestrogen was combined with exercise: bone mass was *increased,* and other symptoms – hot flushes and sleeplessness – improved after three months.

What kind of exercise works for osteoporosis prevention? The slogging peddler on a stationary bike is not doing her bones much good, and swimming doesn't help, according to endocrinologist Dr Bockman, co-director of the Osteoporosis Center at New York's Hospital for Special Surgery. The weight of the body has to be carried by the bones in order to stimulate bone strength. Brisk jogging requires a push-off that is much greater than one's body weight. The point is that one *needs stress* on that hip, and brisk walking can increase that stress in a natural way. 'Everyone can walk briskly,' encourages Dr Bockman. 'Or do serious walking on a treadmill at a tilt, which gives you both weight-bearing and aerobic benefit.' Robert Lindsay's study group at the Helen Hayes Bone Center confirms a measurable prevention of bone loss in postmenopausal women treated with 0.625 mg of Premarin plus Provera. It is not uncommon today to see women started on oestrogen at age sixty or older. It is not too late. 'There is pretty good evidence that giving oestrogen will slow any further bone loss at least up until the age of seventy-five,' says Dr Lindsay. Oestrogen won't reverse the attrition that has already taken place, but it will stop it from getting worse, he adds.

Dr Stanley Birge at Washington University has introduced a radical notion into the debate: 'The effect of oestrogen on protecting against bone fractures may be due to maintaining high mental functioning.' In the OASIS Fall and Hip Fracture Study, women over seventy who were on oestrogen performed better on tasks measuring mental processing speed than women of the same age and education who were not on the hormone. Dr Birge postulates that oestrogen-deprived women over seventy are more likely to suffer the dreaded hip fracture, because when they lose their balance they don't respond fast enough to break their fall. 'Whereas women of the same age who had wrist fractures – evidence they did respond and break their fall – showed twice the mental processing speed.'

Technological advances in machinery now make it possible to measure precisely the weight and strength of a woman's bones. Most major American cities with a medical centre or university have bone densitometer machines (although many are used only for research). Whatever regimen of calcium and exercise and/or hormones a woman tries can be evaluated against her own baseline, to show annually how much bone she is maintaining or losing. It's the same principle as having annual mammograms.

In the UK, however, the situation is quite different. There are only about eighty public machines throughout the country, according to Linda Edwards, and very few of those are available for GP referrals. If one does not live in a major city, it's difficult to get to a machine. But for those women who really want their bone density checked, the National Osteoporosis Society can usually find them a machine and get them on a research programme. Many private facilities have bone densitometer machines available. For a private machine, a woman shouldn't be paying more than about £95–100.

'Physicians have to get used to thinking of bone mass measurement just as they think about a blood pressure measurement,' urges Dr Lindsay. With regard to bone disease in older women, we are exactly where we were with breast cancer twenty years ago: osteoporosis prevention hasn't yet been considered worthy – another example of the scandalous politics of women's health.

HAS ANYONE
SEEN MY MEMORY?

At forty, you can't read the numbers in the telephone book. At fifty, you can't remember them. What's going on?

An even more insidious thief is being quietly noted both by pure-science researchers and by doctors who increasingly hear complaints like those of the very smart best-selling author in Colorado whom I happened to phone one day. 'How are you?' I asked.

'I'm thinking slower – are you? I have tremendous trouble

concentrating. I start to write and just wander. Am I getting stupid?'

All writers have days like this. But this woman, just past fifty, was usually so witty about life's pitfalls. 'What I feel is panic,' she said. 'I tape every interview now, because I know I won't remember. And I'm so intent on remembering, I become extremely irritable. Because if somebody interrupts me while I'm trying to remember, then I'm frightened of losing it.'

She wasn't kidding. 'You feel less competitive, slow off the mark,' she went on. She added glumly, 'I think the bottom line is I'm just plain dimmer.'

Wait a minute, hadn't she been all smiles after having a hysterectomy three years earlier? 'Oh sure, I was just so glad to be finished with cysts and fibroids, and I was mad at all these doctors.' The surgeon told her they had saved one ovary, which should produce enough oestrogen; she wouldn't need to take hormones. That was three years before.

'You might be suffering from oestrogen deprivation,' I said.

'You mean, I'm not stupid, I just need hormones?'

I told her story to Barbara Sherwin, the McGill professor. After the age of forty-eight, she said, that remaining ovary would be quickly withering away. Moreover, manipulation during surgery to remove the uterus often compromises the blood supply to the ovaries. Professor Sherwin said she would be shocked if the writer's oestrogen level wasn't in the post-menopausal range. And the impact on mental acuity can be quite noticeable.

'Something has happened to my memory,' the working women who walk into McGill University Menopause Clinic will often report. They misplace things. It's harder to remember a new phone number, though they always remember the old ones. 'People start getting methodical. They don't just put their glasses down on the kitchen counter, they put them down in a specific spot,' notes Professor Sherwin. Though this temporary strain on short-term memory is quantifiable, the women are not seriously impaired in their daily functioning.

The few studies that show oestrogen loss has a deleterious

effect on mental functioning have been done on surgically menopausal women, where the hormonal drop is sudden and acute. For naturally menopausal women, the effect may be a little fuzzy thinking in the early years of Change of Life. 'When I was in my early fifties, it was impossible for me to look up in an index and hold three different page numbers in my head,' chuckles Canadian newsletter editor O'Leary Cobb. 'I'm fifty-seven now, and it's all come back again. Most of us do recover.'

Oestrogen does help increase the blood flow to the brain. Some women say their memory becomes more acute than ever after they start taking oestrogen. The absence of oestrogen has a powerful effect on synapses at certain sites in the brain, confirms Dr Bruce McEwen, a neuro-endocrinologist at Rockefeller University. He has observed brain chemistry changes in rats during the equivalent of menopause (after their ovaries were removed). 'The number of synaptic connections actually decreases. If you administer oestrogens, these synaptic connections are remade within a few days.' During the female rat's four-day oestrous cycle, which mimics the menstrual cycle, these synapses come and go. As for human females, it has been demonstrated that oestrogens do have an effect on mental functioning – not on IQ but in terms of performance – though Dr McEwen is quick to point out our state of scientific ignorance. 'No one has bothered to look at cognitive behaviour and the effect of oestrogen therapy in a long-term study.' He emphasizes that the subjective experience of cloudy thinking at times during menopause can be equated, for instance, to jet lag: 'It's mostly transient, and certainly reversible.'

Sure enough, when my writer friend from Colorado went to a gynaecologist for her first pelvic exam in four years, the doctor said, 'Your vaginal walls are bone dry.' It was immediately obvious from her age that she needed oestrogen. 'I feel infinitely better, more alert, more moist, more like my old self,' she said. Having overcome her initial resistance to HRT, she now believes she will likely live a longer, healthier life. 'You get on a track – with regular reminders to get mammograms and Pap smears. If something does go wrong, you have an early warning system set up to catch it.'

DANGEROUS BREASTS

Only a year ago the number of women diagnosed with breast cancer was one in ten; now it is one in nine. The breast cancer phobia has now overtaken almost all other health issues surrounding menopause for many women, particularly those who have had a brush with it anywhere in their family. As to why we focus more on women with breast cancer than those with heart disease, Dr Trudy Bush notes that although two thirds of all breast cancers are postmenopausal, one third do occur in younger women, 'so you're thinking of the tragic cases among women forty to fifty-two.'

A woman I'll call Sarah was brutally widowed in her prime of a dashing, beloved, prominent husband. She was left with a lovely apartment and a terrace garden she let go to seed, because she couldn't bear for several years to step out on it and be assaulted by painful memories evoked by the sun and beauty. Sarah was a freelance commercial artist, and a very successful one. But in her misery she soon became blocked creatively and desperately lonely. Then to top it off – hot flushes. Hearing about 'vaginal dryness' from her friends, she wondered if she would lose interest in sex before she had it again. The whole terror of being identified as a menopausal woman overtook her. 'And I'm single, so it matters.'

Off to the plastic surgeon for a full face and neck lift. Then to the gynaecologist for something to 'take away the embarrassment of these drippy hot flushes at dinner parties'. She had to keep herself shelf-fresh – not like some post-dated yogurt – if she was going to keep hope alive for recovering her creativity and her zest for finding a new partner in life.

'But I have these dangerous breasts,' she told me, stroking the unusually large, well-formed bosoms under her T-shirt, as if they had grown alien and were ready at any point to turn on her. 'I have a history of breast cancer among the women in my family.' So, before giving herself hormones she consulted two other doctors, one a reproductive oncologist. Both said, 'Take the hormones. It's worth the benefit.'

'But I admit I did it – do it – with great trepidation. Are you on them? Why? Why don't you get off?' The feverish questioning revealed her frustration and suppressed fears. I talked about my primary concern being prevention of osteoporosis and heart disease – the major dangers for older women. Like a number of my most educated and savvy friends, she didn't know heart disease was the number one killer.

'I also have osteoporosis in my family,' she said miserably. 'So what do I do? I've been on for five years. My doctor never mentioned any end point.'

Doctors seldom do, I said.

'All I know is that once I started taking hormones the flushes stopped and I had a feeling of wellbeing. And I looked okay. All that is important to me, because I'm an older single woman. So my philosophy has been, if it's working, don't mess with it. But am I doing something to my body that I'll kick myself for later?'

She had a bone density test a couple of years before and was told she was fine – the hormones were working. Now she has a new male partner, and she's brought her terrace garden back to life. It's a place of delight where we sat that June day, surrounded by sprouting shrubs and exquisite coral roses, birdsong and cool breeze. 'It gives me such a lift when I wake up to come out here,' Sarah said. She's become a happy, healthy, fully functioning, attractive and sexual woman again. Hormones appear to be integral to her quality of life in her mid-fifties. What risk is she running by taking HRT?

Dr Estelle Ramey points out that the risk of getting breast cancer rises steadily with age, after menopause, in *all* women, including those who are not secreting oestrogen or taking it in replacement hormones – right up to the age of one hundred. Indeed, the single greatest risk factor is age.

Dr Hiram Cody, the New York Hospital breast surgeon, stresses: 'When you're doing a family history, keep in mind that only a first-degree relative – mother or sister – poses an added risk. If it's a grandmother, aunt or cousin, it's not nearly the same added risk, if any risk at all.' Also, to be relevant, one's mother had to have been under the age of fifty when she developed the breast cancer. 'It's a *premenopausal* first-degree relative who contributes a significantly increased risk of breast cancer,' affirms the leading researcher on menopause in Britain, Dr Malcolm Whitehead. 'Even with the worst possible family history,' adds Dr Cody, 'a woman has no more than a fifty-fifty chance of getting breast cancer.'

'What we do know is the one in nine figure,' says Dr Allen. Speaking as a responsible gynaecologist, she recognizes that in prescribing oestrogen to one hundred women, it means that eleven of them will be taking a potential growth stimulus to the breast cancer before it is discovered. 'Whether this changes the long-term prognosis is not known.'

Studies that attempt to document any causative link between HRT and breast cancer are doomed to be inconclusive, because the usual dose of Premarin provides only one quarter of the oestrogen that a woman's fertile ovaries would produce. But it can be said that the more cycles a woman has, naturally and synthetically, the more oestrogen she has in her system over a lifetime.

The primates researcher Kim Wallen points out that for two thousand years most women cycled only two or three times before becoming pregnant, followed by several years of nursing, which again suppressed their period; then they cycled again several times before the next pregnancy. Historically, then, a woman in her reproductive years may have had a total of forty or fifty ovarian cycles. The modern woman may have more than three hundred. 'So human females today are getting a very different pattern of hormonal stimulation,' he concludes. 'Then, when they go through menopause, we are hitting them with another period of exposure to hormones that they never would have had in the past.'

The general world consensus of medical opinion from the best studies is that no evidence suggests there is any danger of increasing the risk of breast cancer by taking HRT for up to five or six years. Quite a number of studies report no danger for possibly up to ten years. There is an increased risk of breast cancer after ten years of use, but exactly what numerical value to put on that increased risk has not been determined. It ranges from 10 to 30 percent. But although there is an increase in the diagnosis of breast cancer after ten years in women on HRT, there is no increase in death from breast cancer. Clinicians postulate it may be because such women are highly aware of their bodies and on a 'wellness track', closely monitored by their physicians.

Another expert emphasizes high-fat diets as the chief culprit in increasing breast cancer rates among American women. Dr Caldwell Esselstyn, Jr., is a maverick surgeon who campaigns for health care 'beyond surgery'. As president of the American Association of Endocrine Surgeons, Dr Esselstyn starts with the data that show nations which consume greater amounts of fat per person have the highest mortality rates of breast cancer. 'And we know that rural Japanese women who still eat a low-fat diet of vegetables, rice and a little fish experience far less breast cancer than Japanese women who have become urbanized and now like steak and french fries,' he says. 'If the lobules and ducts of the breast are constantly being overstimulated by a high fat intake, which leads to higher production of oestrogen, it stands to reason they will be more likely to have cell changes leading to cancer.'

A fatty diet not only adds indirectly to the risk of breast cancer by increasing the oestrogen level; most recently, basic scientists have demonstrated in the laboratory that fat also has a direct effect on tumour growth *independent of oestrogen*. Dr David Rose at the American Health Foundation in Valhalla, New York, injected human female breast cancer cells into two groups of mice. He gave one group a diet of 23 percent corn oil, the same type of fat found in popular margarines. This high-fat diet both increased and accelerated the growth and spread of tumours as compared to the low-fat group. Rose's results, published in the *Journal of the National Cancer Institute* (October, 1991) provide a compelling argument against high-fat diets to protect a woman from *both* heart disease and breast cancer.

'Nobody is arguing against oestrogen supplement for the short-term – the first three to five years of perimenopause and menopause,' says Dr Kuller, the public health expert at the University of Pittsburgh. 'But for the long-term, meaning ten to fifteen years, oestrogen is drug therapy and should only be prescribed for women predisposed to osteoporosis or heart disease, or both.' Dr Kathi Hanna, senior analyst for the Office of Technology Assessment, a research arm of Congress that has surveyed existing studies, agrees: 'It's alarming that practitioners are talking about using hormone therapy indefinitely.'

But here's the rub. The key to hormonal protection against heart disease in older women, according to the Nurses' Study, was that the healthy women were taking oestrogen *currently*. The risks and benefits of oestrogen therapy on eight separate health conditions were toted up in a thorough review by T.M. Mack at the University of Southern California. Stopping treatment with oestrogen at the end of five years would produce a moderate reduction in the expected hospitalizations for breast cancer. But it would also virtually eliminate all the benefits of long-term health enhancement – a Hobson's choice!

But at least we have choices.

SHOULD I
OR SHOULDN'T I?

Women have a right to good, unbiased information about hormone replacement therapy. HRT is a health issue. Most women who take it do not do so to stay youthful and sexy-looking. They take it because they are convinced it is good for their health and wellbeing. They are likely to live longer, more vital lives, and to continue to find the delights of sexuality irresistible.

Other experts I interviewed were emphatically against hormones being given routinely to menopausal women. They remember the mini-epidemic of uterine cancer in the 1970s that followed by several years the celebration of hormone therapy in the book *Feminine Forever*, whose author's foundation was funded in part by three drug companies. That disaster was corrected when doctors began routinely insisting that a woman take cyclical progesterone along with oestrogen. By 1992, a study group convened by Britain's Royal College of Obstetricians and Gynaecologists concluded that the risk of uterine cancer is virtually eliminated by using a progesterone. But given this history, the credibility of experts is not very high with women.

At least two recent American presidents have been on hormone replacement therapy. John Kennedy's adrenal glands were almost completely deteriorated. (Without the regulatory hormones the adrenals produce, wasting and death is the end result.) Even as he campaigned in the watershed 1960 election against Richard Nixon, Kennedy's hormonal condition was kept under control by replacement hormones. A wall of denial and cover stories kept his adrenal insufficiency and HRT regimen secret for many years, the silence being broken only in 1992 by two pathologists who conducted his autopsy.

Similarly, the public didn't know that President George Bush had started hormone replacement therapy when he began acting jittery in the summer of 1991. The public puzzled over the manic energy he displayed, racing around in his cigarette boat and jumping from one sport to another, all the while he was calling together a worldwide military response to Saddam Hussein's invasion of Kuwait. The White House doctor eventually disclosed that the President's overactive thyroid gland had been treated with radioactive iodine and destroyed in April 1991, and that he must take a daily dose of the hormone that his body no longer makes naturally. The thyroid hormone is a major regulator of the body's metabolism. Its functions can be easily maintained by taking the hormone, but the body is highly sensitive to dosages, and chronic stress or heavy travel with changing of time zones can throw everything off. Thus, when Bush began behaving erratically and making constant verbal gaffes in his speeches at the height of his summer '92 re-election campaign, a wave of rumours about his health flooded the stock market. The crisis prompted his doctor, Burton Lee, to disclose to the press that he had recently been 'messing around' with Bush's dosage of hormone replacement.

So, even world leaders can have volatile hormones.

Dr Nita Nelson, a Los Angeles gynaecologist, makes the case that oestrogen is the only hormone that people are asked to live without. 'If a woman is diabetic and doesn't have enough insulin, we don't say, 'Try to live without the insulin.' We know she's going to die sooner and that the years she has left will be poor unless we replace the insulin she's missing. The same goes for thyroid deficiencies. Oestrogen is the only one we ask women to do without.'

So persuasive is the evidence of the multiple protective benefits of oestrogen, many experts are now openly promoting oestrogen replacement therapy. I asked one of the major researchers in Europe, Dr Malcolm Whitehead, director of the menopause clinic at Kings College Hospital in London and president of the International Menopause Society, 'If it was your wife, what would you tell her about coming to a decision?'

'I don't see it as much of a conundrum, perhaps because I'm a man,' he opines. 'If oestrogens really do reduce coronary-artery disease death by fifty percent, that factor alone will swamp any other factor in the equation.' Dr Whitehead openly envies women for *having* a choice – men don't. 'We are stuck from the time we're born to the time we die with arterial disease as a sword of Damocles hanging over us.'

Some top researchers are even reversing themselves on the conventional prescription for *combined* hormone replacement therapy. The synthetic progesterones continue to present a problem. The best data from the United Kingdom (by Roger King and Tom Anderson at the Imperial Cancer Research Fund) indicate that the effect of progestins on breast tissue is either neutral or may slightly increase the risk of cell division. 'One would predict that, because women get lumpy breasts before their period when progesterone is at a high level in the bloodstream,' affirms Dr Whitehead.

The reason to use a progesterone is to protect the uterus. Oestrogen used alone has been clearly linked with an increased incidence of uterine cancer. Abnormal bleeding patterns may be able to warn early of precancerous changes in the lining of the uterus. However, this early sign does not always occur, warns Dr Allen. Fortunately, the uterine lining is not difficult to monitor. Endometrial biopsy and/or a D&C are useful and easily performed. Recent findings suggest that ultrasound may be able to monitor the uterine lining as well. There is a high cure rate with uterine cancer that is caught early.

Dr Robert Lindsay, the osteoporosis expert, is not an enthusiastic supporter of progestins. 'If you give 10 mg of Provera in combination with the Premarin, many women feel premenstrual and crabby and irritable. They call up and say, "Why did you give me that stuff?" The concern is that many people who would gain in healthy active years, on oestrogen replacement, are turned off by the required addition of a progestin and the continuation of periods.'

The continuation of periods is the main reason women give for discontinuing hormones. American doctors are now solving this problem by giving their patients a synthetic progesterone only every few months. Or a woman takes a smaller amount of the progesterone every day along with the oestrogen, for 25 days. It smoothes out her cycle, she doesn't have storms of hormonal highs and lows, and after six months at most, periods generally cease. 'In some women that works very well, but we don't really know yet if it reduces or eliminates the risk of uterine cancer,' adds Dr Lindsay.

There are now at least a dozen different regimens recommended by doctors for combining oestrogen and a progesterone. No two women respond the same way. 'I always tell people the first year is trial and error,' says Barbara Sherwin at the McGill University clinic. 'We're constantly readjusting the dose, the types of products, and the regimen.' In Britain, it is very common for a woman to take HRT for a few months and then go off it because of unpleasant side effects, not realizing that there are other alternative dosages and regimens with which she can experiment.

A new way of administering the counter-hormone is progesterone in an oral micronized form, which is the only way the body can absorb the *natural* hormone. The progesterone in this product comes from either the South American yam or the soybean plant. 'It doesn't have all the negative side effects of Provera but many of the positive effects you're looking for from a progesterone,' enthuses Dr Jamie Grifo, a new-generation gynaecologist at New York Hospital. He and Dr Notelovitz in Gainesville believe oral micronized natural progesterone is the wave of the future. A study on twelve women with moderate to severe menopausal symptoms by Dr Joel T. Hargrove at Vanderbilt University Medical Center tested the safety of a daily combination of natural oral micronized progesterone (200–300 mg) with oestrogen. After six months, the combination improved symptoms with minimal side effects and left the women with a thin endometrium and no evidence of suspicious changes in tissue. Also, withdrawal bleeding stopped. It also raised the good cholesterol (thereby eliminating the counterproductive effects of synthetic progestins on the heart disease protection offered by oestrogen).

The British expert, Dr Whitehead, is not so optimistic about oral micronized progesterone (OMP). 'In our experience OMP causes sleepiness and lassitude when given in dosage high enough to ensure endometrial protection.' (In a dose-ranging study he did at Kings College Hospital, only 300 mg of OMP a day for ten days was sufficient to reproduce the effect of the body's own progesterone during the luteal phase of the menstrual cycle. Although a 200 mg daily dose does suppress cell duplication, it does not produce the full secretory transformation of the uterine lining.)

'What does a woman do then, if the only dose that protects her makes her fall asleep?' I asked Dr Whitehead.

'Then you have a problem.'

Acknowledging the problem, Meir Stampfer, the principal investigator on the Nurses' Study of heart disease, writes, 'An important challenge is to develop a progestin regimen or formulation that will maintain protection of the uterus, yet not impair the benefits of oestrogen on lipids.'

The British and Europeans have more progestin agents available than do American physicians. Dr Whitehead favours a Dutch-made agent, derived from the natural progesterone, called Duphaston, made by Duphar in Holland and licensed for use in the United Kingdom. 'It gives you good protection of the uterus but, in our experience, it causes few adverse symptomatic and psychological effects and gives you little of the reduction in cardioprotective effect.'

Here is a guide to the different preparations available in Europe. If one doesn't suit a woman, a different chemical formulation likely will.

Premarin and *Oestradiol* are the most commonly used forms of oestrogen.

The *Estraderm patch* is an increasingly popular method of delivering oestrogen to the body. A small adhesive bandage releases the hormone through the skin, with the advantage that it maintains a continuous, consistent level of oestrogen in the system, like a time-release capsule. It is not metabolized through the liver and therefore has no impact on digestive diseases. The United States drug regulatory agency recently approved Estraderm as a treatment for menopause and osteo-porosis. Oestrogen delivered in this form, however, has not proven to be as beneficial in protecting against heart disease as oestrogen taken orally.

Besides *Provera*, there are synthetic progestins available in Europe that one can't get in the United States.

Duphaston, a unique compound, is very similar to natural pro-gesterone. The only difference between it and the natural pro-gesterone form is that a group of atoms, above and below the plane of the molecule, are reversed in position. It is the best tolerated of all the progestogens. In a study which was published in the *British Journal of Obstetrics and Gynaecology* a few years ago, says Dr John Moran, 'it was proved to be more or less lipid-neutral, with no significant effect on total cholesterol, LDL or HDL.'

Norathindrone is prescribed for women who have side effects with Provera and Duphaston. It's a C-19 nortestosterone derivative. While it doesn't have testosterone in it, it does have male hormone-like side effects.

Norgestrel, also a C-19 nortestosterone derivative, is even more potent.

There is also a natural progesterone available which can be given either as a suppository or as a vaginal pessary, thereby avoiding the intestinal system to get right into circulation.

There are two basic HRT regimens. The standard preparation given by the National Health Service in the UK is *Prempak.* Basically it is Premarin available in two strengths, 0.625 mg or 1.25 mg. It provides a continuous oestrogen throughout the 28-day calendar, but for the last twelve days it administers a small dose of the progestogen. Sometimes it's called Prempak-C. The 'C' just means continuous.

The second means of delivering HRT combines oestrogenic and progestogenic properties with a small testosterone effect. *Livial* (also called tibolone) is effective in alleviating menopausal symptoms and may also help to protect against osteoporosis. There is no monthly bleed. It's a derivative of a C-19 progestogen. The hitch is that it can only be given to a limited group of women. First, a woman must be strictly postmenopausal. If a perimenopausal woman were to take Livial, the underlying cycle would break through to cause bleeding. Acne is also a frequent side effect. And because its properties are predominantly progestogenic, it's not recommended for someone who has developed PMS, because she would be likely to have PMS all the time on Livial.

The debate over 'natural' vs. 'medicalized' menopause will only grow more vigorous as boomers come along. I was asked to give a talk in San Diego to women state legislators from all over the country on the subject of menopause. It was quite amazing: four hundred busy political women stayed for several hours, on the last Sunday of their conference, to discuss every aspect of the Change. Many of them came to microphones to describe their experiences. Finally, Betty Friedan took her turn and poo-pooed the whole subject. Hormones were dangerous, and besides, who needs them? Drawing only on her own experience, she shrugged, 'I *may* have had a hot flush, one hot flush, while I was giving a major speech in the middle of the Seventies.'

But no woman's genetic makeup should be held up as the model for abstinence from hormones, making the next woman feel lesser for having a different nervous system, different metabolism, and different stores of hormones, just as she has different depths of pigment and strands of DNA in the tangle of her own creation.

'We wear glasses when our eyes are bad, we use hearing aids, we get false teeth, and now we're putting in new knees and hips,' counters Columbia University physiologist Fredi Kronenberg, a researcher in rehabilitation medicine at Columbia University, Hospital of Physicians and Surgeons. 'Oestrogen affects our hearts, our minds, our bones, our behaviour and our sexual function and desire.' Her basic argument is how can women expect to live thirty-five more years and *not* supplement the oestrogen they no longer make naturally?

Several studies indicate that women live longer if they are on oestrogen, notably the Leisure World Study of 8,881 women aged forty to one hundred and one in a southern California retirement community. The women completed a health survey in 1981 and were followed up seven years later. 20 percent fewer of the women with a history of oestrogen use had died from any cause, compared with those who had never taken oestrogen. The more startling evidence reported in 1991 is that the longer the women used oestrogen replacement therapy, the lower was their mortality risk. Current users who had taken oestrogen for more than fifteen years enjoyed twice the benefit – a 40 percent reduction – in their overall mortality.

'Women with symptoms certainly feel better when they

take oestrogen, and those in professional positions almost always feel they work and concentrate better,' concludes Dr Lindsay. The standard comment volunteered by British women who have been on long-term hormone replacement therapy, according to Dr Whitehead, is 'They say they feel fit and they always seem to have four times as much energy as their neighbours do.'

To make it easy for your doctor to take care of you during these years, know what you want. Here are questions to ask yourself:

- Is there any evidence of osteoporosis in your family?
- Did your mother or a sister have breast cancer? How young? Was it oestrogen-sensitive?
- Is there any family history of heart disease?
- Is there a family history of cancer of the uterus?
- Did you have serious PMS?
- How long have you been perimenopausal? (The longer it takes you to move from irregular cycles to no cycles, the more likely you are to have physical and emotional symptoms.)
- Rank order, on a scale of one to ten, what concerns you most about menopause; i.e. No. 1 might be the embarrassment of hot flushes in public, and No. 10 might be the fear of breast cancer or of losing memory and concentration.

Victims of breast cancer are doubly deprived. Until recently, it has been considered *verboten* to give hormone replacement therapy to postmenopausal women with breast cancer. Today, for women with a terribly symptomatic menopause adding to their depression over losing a breast, the 'quality of life' issue must by weighed in the balance. Especially if they have had a hysterectomy, and have no circulating hormones at all, they may feel life is hardly worth living. Some physicians now offer them the choice of taking a short course of HRT.

'We've prescribed for a small series of postmenopausal patients with breast cancer oestrogen plus a low dose of pro-gesterone – *given continuously, together, every single day*, without break for three to six months,' describes Dr Basil Stoll, an oncologist at St Thomas's Hospital in London. The most important part, he underlines, is the continuous delivery of the progesterone, which also alleviates a withdrawal bleed. 'The patient's symptoms are relieved and there is no evidence that their risk of breast cancer is increased.' The short course, he says, is usually enough to carry the woman over the peak of hot flushes. The number of patients in his series is only fifteen, and they have been followed up for only two years. They have had no recurrence of cancer.

If you have had a precancerous condition in the cervix, not to worry; cervical cancer is not hormone-dependent. Also, there is no evidence that oestrogen increases the risk of ovarian cancer.

COST-BENEFITS OF HORMONE REPLACEMENT THERAPY

Risks	*Benefits*
1. Possible increased risk of cancer of uterus	1. Prevents osteoporosis
2. Unknown associations with breast cancer	2. Decreases heart attacks
3. Continued menstruation possible	3. No hot flushes
4. Breast swelling or pain	4. Decreases insomnia
5. Premenstrual-like syndrome on progesterone	5. Improves energy
6. Expense of doctors' visits and tests for screening	6. Improves mood and sense of wellbeing
	7. Restores sexual interest and comfort
	8. May improve concentration and memory
	9. May improve longevity

DO I HAVE
TO STAY ON
HORMONES FOR EVER?

One of the scare statements often repeated is that hormones will only put off the inevitable. 'A woman who starts on hormones will have to stay on for ever because if she stops, all the menopausal symptoms will return with a vengeance,' a prominent New York gynaecologist told a new patient. This 'express train' scenario is false, says Dr Lila A. Wallis, a New York internist with forty years of clinical experience. Many older patients have grown into their sixties under her care as users of hormone replacement therapy.

'In the very early menopause, women require larger doses of oestrogens in order to control their symptoms,' says Dr Wallis. 'As they get older, the oestrogens can be cut down and the patient is more tolerant of the decreased dose.'

The one action to avoid is to go off hormones 'cold turkey'. The operative generalization is this: *The more abrupt the drop in oestrogen, the more severe are the symptoms.* This explains the severity of symptoms often reported after a hysterectomy, or during a sudden, stress-related menopause, just as it explains the flare-up of symptoms that may occur if a woman who's been suppressing them for a decade with HRT abruptly discontinues the hormone bath to which the body is accustomed. There is a simple way to avoid this problem: tapering off. Dr Wallis advises her older patients to watch the 'pause' at the end of the month and note whether or not hot flushes or any other symptoms resurface. As symptoms subside, the regimen of replacement hormones can be gradually reduced. The body is allowed to adjust over time.

HELP IS
ON THE WAY

The politics of menopause are at last being challenged by female health professionals and lawmakers. What can you do?

We can all help to break the conspiracy of silence about menopause by starting self-help groups and sending out educational messages in every way, shape and form. We will render normalcy to a normal transition only by talking about it, and sharing what we do know and what we are determined to find out.

If we approach this journey with optimism, determined to become informed consumers of health information, and choosy about the physician who will work with us as a partner in managing a natural life transition rather than expecting a compliant 'patient', most of us can live and love and work and cope quite well. Here are three important ways to think about the passage through menopause:

First, consider the time you have left to live – one half of your *adult* life. If you have the good fortune to reach menopause, you have a responsibility to educate yourself on how to preserve your physical and mental wellbeing so that your older years can be vigorous and independent. Think of going for the long haul. Take a life review of where you have been, the parts of yourself you have already lived out, and those yearnings you left behind as a girl. How can you put play back into your life? How can you turn your talents and life skills to caregiving in the broader, even worldly sphere? What adventure of mind or heart or bold personal challenge would your ideal future self dare to take? Consult her, then follow her lead!

Second, find the information you need to help you manage your menopausal transition. A woman's wellness centre may be sufficient to answer your questions. Most doctors will tell you if you ask them honestly: how many women do you treat over the age of forty-five? (That will tell you how interested or experienced the physician is in treating menopause.) Ask the doctor to describe menopause to you. Then ask questions. If your inquiries are brushed off with pat or curt answers, walk away. There is no clear menopausal test. If you want some hormonal guidelines, the tests to ask for are your oestrogen level and LH and FSH levels and an osteoporosis screening. But your best guide is your own symptoms.

Be an inquiring, even challenging, partner, not a passive follower of doctor-as-God. Decisions on how to plan for the health and wellbeing of your next thirty years or more cannot be made in a twenty-minute visit to your doctor, any more than you would decide on the purchase of an expensive car in that time. Expect a year of trial and error.

Third, take charge of the transformation. That means becoming serious about regular exercise. Find something you like to do: best if it requires making an appointment or a social date because then you'll have to keep to it; but you can also park at the end of the mall and walk briskly with march music on your Walkman. This physical effort will support your bones, heart, lungs, as it pumps oxygen for clear thinking and endorphins for good feeling straight to your brain. Transformation also means looking for ways to stop pushing yourself so hard professionally or inviting so much stress. It may help to find a therapist or a group to work with in identifying the woman you want to be for the rest of your life.

Finally, this momentous passage invites meditation and spiritual exploration. A wise woman will make time to contemplate things eternal and appreciate the life she has.

Coalescence

Once the ovarian transition is complete, a woman enters a new state of equilibrium. Her energy, moods, and overall sense of physical and mental wellbeing should be restored, but with a difference. Think of it as discarding the shell of the reproductive self – who came into being in adolescence – and coming out the other side to *coalescence*. (*Coalesce* means to come together, to unite; *-escence* denotes action or process, a change state.)

It is a time when all the wisdom a woman has gathered from fifty years of experience in living comes together. Once she is no longer confined to the culture's definition of woman as a primarily sexual object and breeder, a full unity of her feminine and masculine sides is possible. As she moves beyond gender definition, she gains new licence to speak her mind and initiate action.

The time sense changes. People in their late thirties and early forties are commonly pursued by a frantic hurry-up feeling – as if everything they have missed out on must be seized immediately, or lost for ever. This midlife agitation is often revived for women by the perimenopausal panic in the mid to late forties. As suggested, the foreshortening of time sense takes place because the forties represent the old age of youth, while the fifties open up the youth of Second Adulthood. What may have been seen as a dead end is now perceptible as a gateway to years ahead that spread out like a brand new playing field.

'I spent a large part of my early adult life on logistics – just getting from point A to point B with three young children and no money,' said an animated 59-year-old schoolteacher, describing her postmenopausal change of outlook. 'Now, with no responsibilities, with three functioning children who are off on their own, it's a liberation that is difficult to explain . . . it's emotional, physical, financial – total.'

We have a second chance in postmenopause, unencumbered by the day-to-day caregiving and thousand and one details of feeling that most women pour into the long parental emergency, to focus on the things we most love and to redirect our creativity in the most individual of ways. We must make an alliance with our changing bodies and negotiate with our vanity. No, we are never again going to be that girl of our idealized inner eye. The task now is to find a new 'future self' in whom we can invest our trust and enthusiasm.

Today's 'coalescents' are mapping out a whole new stage of life. Despite all the idiosyncrasies of this age group, common refrains emerged in the stories given by American women in their fifties:

'Making choices is so much easier,' was a comment echoed from coast to coast.

'You don't get your period *and* you don't have to panic when you don't,' summed up a West Coast woman.

'You don't have to play the girl game any more,' said an attractive divorcée who's let her hair go grey. 'But it's still all right to be a vulnerable female person and allow yourself moments of weakness. Now it's *your* choice.'

The 'empty nest', which we were told by psychoanalytic theorists would leave us feeling useless and lacking in self-concept, turns out not to register as a main concern in large-scale contemporary studies. When women mentioned it at all in interviews with me, it was usually with relief or relish.

'After being liberated from keeping those five long-legged sons filled up, a new world opened up to me as I approached fifty,' said a Southern woman who had happily fulfilled the duties of a full-time wife. 'One of the kids said, "Mom, what

are you going to do with yourself, now that we're all gone?"
I said, "Hon, I don't know, but count on it – I'm going to have
fun!"'

'The freedom of middle age is fantastic!' exulted a former
homemaker who loves her new life as a real estate agent.
'Now *Mom* can lie down before dinner. Or I can pay somebody
else to do dinner. Or I don't have to have dinner at all.'

'Watch out, I'm heading down hill and I'm on a roll!' called
a Colorado woman as she passed me on the jogging track.

A great discovery of the fifties is the *courage to go against*
– against conformist behaviour and conventional wisdom. A
woman can at last integrate the rebellious boy in herself, left
behind back when she was ten or eleven and eager for adventure and before she became vulnerable, i.e, capable of being
violated. Social psychologist Bernice Neugarten reports that
as women move into later life, they become more accepting
of their own aggressive and egocentric impulses, and feel less
guilty. Research on female cognition has demonstrated that
women shift more fluidly than men from intellect to intuition,
or from linear to non-linear thinking, seeing the events of life
less as black and white than as a continuum. Given the added
status and confidence of the postmenopausal state, women are
in an optimum position to voice their convictions and make a
powerful public impact. An initial sense of timidity and danger
may give way to relief and excitement, as the new older
women realize there are still many 'firsts' ahead. Once they
stop clinging to a life and conditions that have been outgrown,
they can stake out their freedom at last. This usually happens
by the mid-fifties, as is evident in the following excerpts from
interviews:

'I'm not pulling my punches like I used to – I'm saying more
of the things I really think,' boasted a beautiful Rochester
woman, now sixty-eight, who has remade herself into an
organizational management executive.

'I grew up mechanical, I could fix a flat or repair the roof,
but I always deferred,' admitted a well-built African-American

woman of sixty who takes care of a three-family house. 'Now
I don't need anybody to tell me how.'

'You have the whole spectrum of intellectual capacity to
draw on,' enthused a physician who left conventional medicine
and is enlivened in her late fifties by practising nutritional
medicine.

Such comments hint at the welcome change of perspective as
women come through the disequilibrium of menopause into
the stage of mastery that follows it – a passage that is not
cause for remorse but for celebration. In fact, my previous
studies of life stages on sixty thousand adult Americans established that women in their fifties, by self-report, had a greater
sense of wellbeing than at any previous stage in their lives. A
considerable body of psychological study data has accumu-
lated since then confirming that women are least likely to be
clinically depressed in middle age.

EXTRA-SEXUAL
PASSIONS

At a small conference on 'The New Older Woman', organized
by Group Four, a consulting partnership, and held at the
Esalen Institute in summer '91, prominent American women
from diverse backgrounds and professions were invited to
share viewpoints on what it's like to be energetic, ambitious,
optimistic, and over fifty in today's America. Most said they
had negotiated the passage through menopause with a minimum of difficulty. The happy little secret they shared was that
they had enjoyed the best sex of their lives during and just
after menopause, between the ages of forty-five and fifty-five.
(Granted, their generation had been sexually repressed in

youth.) These were also women of a generation totally unschooled in what to expect of menopause. The usual comment was that they were 'too busy' with career, personal relationships or family to dwell on the physical or psychological accompaniments to the Change of Life.

Participants now in their sixties or older agreed that there came a point, sometime in their fifties, when they had to let go of – or at least stop trying to hang on to – their youthful image, and move on. Although painful at the time, they had all found a source of new vitality and exhilaration – a 'kicker'. As each one described her personal struggle, a common denominator emerged and the group hit upon something profound:

The source of continuing aliveness was to find your passion and pursue it, with whole heart and single mind. It is essential to *claim the pause* and find this new source of aliveness and meaning that will make the years ahead even more precious than those past.

For several of the women the passion was to correct an ignored community or societal wrong: Harriet Woods, for example, the former lieutenant governor of Missouri, had lost a Senate race and turned to creating a brand new political institution, a think tank at the University of Missouri. She went on to become president of the National Women's Political Caucus, the only bipartisan national membership organization that recruits, trains and supports women for elective and appointive office. In both roles she pursues her passion: to help women learn to use power in ways different from hierarchical, victimizing male models, with an eye to transforming society. 'Age no longer has the same relevance it used to have,' she affirms. 'Whether it is through caregiving or creating new institutions as I just did ... it happens for women who are beyond what was once thought of as the curve for making a contribution.'

Others had found more private passions: going back to college to finish a degree, writing a book, or the pursuit of knowledge in a special field for the pure pleasure of knowing.

It was agreed that the older woman with fewer resources

often feels isolated, even cheated. Just as she feels free to pursue personal goals, her husband may be going into decline or physical dependency; returning children may try to manipulate her into remaining chief cook and laundrywoman; divorce or ailing parents may cramp her financially. But although these realities might sound like arguments against risk-taking at this time of life, in fact they make it all the more essential to dare new explorations.

How – or if – one *welcomes* postmenopause, and consciously prepares for the new freedom it offers, makes all the difference in reaping the benefits of the stages beyond. The gateway to our Second Adulthood is a passage to be approached with pleasurable anticipation, as we take control over our lives and assume the new licence to be outrageous. Anthropologist Catherine Bateson counsels: 'Say to yourself, I'm going to start a new life. It could be a stage of expansiveness or withdrawal. It could be a time of introversion or of worldly adventure.'

'Age rage,' as psychologist Ellen McGrath describes it in her new book on healthy depressions, *When Feeling Bad is Good*, is a predictable response to the downgrading that older women (and men) experience in most Western societies today. But a healthy depression is only transitional, until one moves through the passage and transforms old patterns of thinking and acting.

The key to finding a new sense of empowerment in the Second Adulthood comes from moving through the crisis of ageing to *generativity*. This entails a profound shift from pouring all one's energies into procreation or raising one's immediate children, or into one's own advancement, towards feeling a voluntary obligation to care for others in a larger sense.

There is a natural generative role into which the postmenopausal woman comfortably fits, going back to prehistory. It is that of the matriarch. The historical biographer, Antonia Fraser, revels in this role. 'People *love* women who have had lots of children,' she purrs (she has had six). 'When one says, "I'm about to have my fourth grandchild and the fifth is on the way," people say, "Oh, isn't that wonderful?" It makes them feel *tribally* good. Everybody feels more comfortable with a matriarch than a patriarch.'

Antonia Fraser takes strong issue with Germaine Greer's view that women after menopause are seen as null and void and so should welcome sterility and relax into celibacy. 'You can't regard all women in menopause as the same,' she warns. 'There is a grand division between those who have had children and those who haven't.'

The childless Greer has revealed in interviews over the years an absence of intimacy in her life. Today she lives alone in a country farmhouse, claiming celibacy to be her preference. Having always, as she says, 'been principally interested in men for sex,' the concept of an intimate *relationship* with a man of the sort that creates almost a third being – a mutuality between husbands and wives that is only enriched by growing older together – is apparently not within her comprehension. In a striking self-revelation, she writes in *The Change*, 'If you haven't managed to get a husband, let alone keep him alive and by your side until you are fifty, if you haven't borne any children or have been unable to get the ones you have brought up to treat you decently . . . then you'll probably make a hash of the menopause.'

In preparing for a smooth postmenopausal passage, it is useful to look to the most vital women of later age and how they have met the challenges of later-life passages. Cecelia Hurwich, a PhD candidate in later life developmental psychology, did a ten-year longitudinal study on *Vital Women in Their Eighties and Nineties* at the Center for Psychological Studies at Berkeley. The women she studied had remained active and creative through unusually productive Second Adulthoods and well into old age. They all prized a nonconformist state of mind; they had mastered the art of 'letting go' gracefully of some things so they could give their attention to fine-tuned priorities; they continued to live in their own homes and kept up with community or worldly projects that had always been of interest to them; and they retained close contact with nature and a multigenerational network of friends.

The sense of danger vs. safeness is another dimension that changes dramatically in the postmenopause stages. Women in the Hurwich study said the worst of their fears of ageing and death had been addressed, and laid to rest, while they were in their fifties – and after that these negative concerns were increasingly discarded. Even those who were widowed or divorced had found love – and lovers – through sharing the most natural of pleasures: music, gardening, walking, travelling; and several spoke enthusiastically of having active and satisfying sex lives. One woman, asked how she felt about the automatic assumption that women in their seventies and eighties lost all interest in sex, answered after a long pause: 'This is how it is for me. I've become a vegetarian, but every once in a while I want a piece of steak. And I go out and get it and eat it and enjoy it.'

WISEWOMAN POWER

Women who no longer belong to somebody now can belong to everybody – the community, a chosen circle of friends, a worship group, or even the world – by virtue of contributing knowledge or creative insight or healing gifts. In fact, the elder women who survived in ancient or tribal cultures developed a way to further species survival *independent* of their wombs. These women became sources of experience and wisdom and were often venerated as shamans with healing powers, upon whom both individuals and tribe depended to handle crises. As the influence of female deities increased steadily up to about 500 BC, the role of medicine man was assumed by medicine woman. 'The fact that women were shamans during this period indicates they had entered into the most authoritative and honoured ranks of healers,' writes Jeanne Achterberg in *Woman As Healer.*

Wisdom, or the collective practical knowledge of the culture that is more simply termed common sense, has continued up through history to be associated with older women. Even in premodern times, when Christianity rejected females as deities or primary healers, great public women did emerge and exert their influence through the religious system. Some became prized as advisors to emperors and popes, turned to for their healing powers, venerated as holy – and it turns out that they were usually near fifty when they took on this aura of wisewomen.

Today's pioneering women in postmenopause in advanced societies eventually give up the futile gallantry of trying to remain the same younger self. Coming through the passage of menopause they reach a new plateau of contentment and self-acceptance, along with a broader view of the world that not only enriches one's individual personality but gives one a new perspective on life and humankind. Such women – there are more and more of them today – find a potent new burst of energy by their mid-fifties.

Margaret Mead spoke frequently about postmenopausal zest and regarded it as a widespread phenomenon. When Mary Catherine Bateson was writing her own book, *Composing a Life*, she was unable to find a formal discussion of the phenomenon mentioned by her mother. Yet Dr Mead certainly experienced a grand bloom in her fifties, following on a shattering series of blows in her forties.

When the bomb exploded over Hiroshima, Mead tore up every page of a book she had nearly finished. As she wrote in her autobiography, *Blackberry Winter*, 'Every sentence was out of date. We had entered a new age. My years as a collaborating wife . . . also came to an end.' She was forty-three. Her adored husband left the marriage, her closest colleague died, and she spent several years devising a new way of working without them, while improvising a life as a divorced professional mother of a small child.

But between the ages of forty-five and fifty-five, as Bateson pieces together the famous anthropologist's history, 'she seemed to become prettier, she bought a couple of designer dresses for the first time, from Fabiani, and I think she started a new romantic relationship. Without question, she went through a complete professional renaissance.' Boldly, Dr Mead decided to return to the field at the age of fifty-one. She boned up on languages she had learned twenty years before, and went back to New Guinea, forging a major intellectual new start with groundbreaking research on social change published in the book *New Lives For Old*.

In fact, hormonal changes may partly explain why so many women describe a vastly increased store of energy after menopause, while some men move towards despair and decline. A good deal of the energy of a younger woman goes into producing enough of the hormone progesterone to sustain a possible pregnancy. Postmenopausal women no longer suffer from the handicap of continually fluctuating levels of progesterone. Menopause also puts an end to the mood swings of the menstrual years.

Middle-aged men have no such abrupt shutdown of hormone production, and no accompanying surge of energy. 'In my view, it's not so much that men decline, but that women start to overtake them,' posits Dr Katharina Dalton, a leading British endocrinologist. 'It is also a medical fact that men's bodies age far faster than women's ... Middle-aged men do not experience the new lease of life, the sense of liberation that postmenopausal women often enjoy. Their health gets worse, while that of their wives gets better.'

This fact places many middle-aged wives in the role of woman-as-healer. They don't have to have the status of a prehistoric medicine woman or that of a medieval abbess to tap into their postmenopausal powers of active imagination, whereby they may be able to lead a seriously ill spouse or parent towards self-healing or spiritual comfort.

There is even a hormonal explanation to underscore the observation across cultures of the switch in male-female behaviour during middle age, a phenomenon I've called the 'sexual diamond'. From their mid-forties to their sixties, women tend to become more aggressive and goal-oriented, while men show a tender and vulnerable side that may have been formerly suppressed. Women whose ovaries have stopped putting out the female sex hormone, oestrogen, still produce in the cortex of their ovaries a small but consistent amount of the male sex hormone, testosterone. The relatively high level of testosterone in about fifty percent of postmenopausal females could partially explain the take-charge behaviour so often exhibited by middle-aged women. Meanwhile, men's testosterone levels are gradually decreasing with age, while they continue to produce a relatively stable amount of oestrogen. They may be going through their own version of 'male menopause'. A crisis of potency, it may be cued by relatively slight changes in sexual prowess, but it is primarily a psychological confrontation with what it means to be a man as physical strength ebbs. Many men in their fifties shift to a lower gear, while their wives and female contemporaries accelerate, fuelled by their new postmenopausal energy and self-assertiveness.

'Do you know how you feel a week after your period ends – like you could climb mountains and slay dragons? That's how a postmenopausal woman feels all the time, if she's conscious of it,' says Elizabeth Stevenson, a Jungian analyst in Cambridge.

Stevenson had a year of hot flushes, which she relieved with acupuncture, and by the age of fifty-two broke through to a state of postmenopausal zest. 'It's both physical and psychological,' she says. Now fifty-five, she doesn't have the same energy level she had at twenty-five, but she monitors and shepherds her energy so that her working days begin at eight and end at eight. If she eats right and exercises, she says, the consciousness of the wisewoman is always with her.

EMPTYING AND REFILLING

Mastering the physical and psychological challenges of the Change might be seen as a test, a necessary exercise, forcing us to look ahead and accept the new perspective coming into view. Each major life passage entails emptying and refilling. It is particularly literal, and poignant, during menopause. There is first the gushing, like the reddening of a tree as it blazes out in autumn with a flaming canopy before going dormant. As we move into postmenopause, we are emptied of the menses that have dominated our reproductive phase. We are reduced to basics, forced to lie fallow. Within that emptiness, watered by tears over the surrender of our magical powers of birthing, if we hold fast through the dark night of unknowing, we can discover our greater fertility. Contemplating the face of nature reminds us of our responsibility for creation and protection of the earth, and of earth wisdom. While men are programmed by evolution to live short, high-performance lives, women are wired to endure.

The greatest boon of menopause is that it forces us to tune in to our body's needs and quirks, and to stay intimately tuned. It is, after all, the house in which we will dwell for the rest of our days, and we will be comfortable in it only if we learn how to turn down the stress on our heart and keep the mineral turning over in our bone. A new balance must be struck between output and input. What is needed for replenishment? For some women it's the decision to take off a four-day weekend every six weeks – to climb a mountain, look at the sea, or simply drop out with music or books – whatever it takes to empty one's cares and find the calm for centring. For others, the Change is the signal to change unhealthy eating habits, stop smoking, invest in serious exercise and learn what their body needs to feel good. For those who are already exercise habitués, they may need to balance aerobic exercise, which is demanding of the body, with yoga or meditation.

But more than that, of all the passages, the Change of Life is a process of emptying and refilling that requires a new companionship between mind and body.

I wasn't ready to be fifty until I was fifty-two. By then, I had made several logical steps up to a new perspective. If we allow the mind to expand and explore higher realities, the body follows. At some point over the course of those two years I suddenly knew, with utter certainty, that as I grew older I was going to get better. I invited my body to accept that new reality. I could begin to visualize, positively, the vast unmarked territory from here to my eighties. The journey excited me. I felt, almost giddily, like a pioneer. And by then, I had sorted out the practical aids and rituals that belonged in my long-term survival kit.

My personal choice, predicated on a family history of severe osteoporosis and no cancer, is to use hormone replacement therapy. It took me, however, a couple of years of experimentation before I found the right preparations and regimen to complement the peculiarities of my body chemistry. I am very glad I had the patience to stick it out. I find the patch works very conveniently to deliver an even, sustained amount of oestrogen. Being among that one third of women who find the standard synthetic progesterone hard to tolerate, I was pleased to discover a newer drug, Duphaston, that mimics the natural progesterone produced by the body in all but the position of a single molecule. I heard about it in my interviews with Dr John Moran and Dr Mike Ellerington in London, both of whom found their patients enthusiastic about it. Produced by a Dutch company, it is available in the UK and Europe, though it is not expected to be available in the United States for another five years. But hormones are only a part of the survival kit.

Having systematically researched how to stem the crumbling wherever I could, without surgery or making a fool of myself, I decided to let myself gain a little weight – it's called 'sacrificing the fanny for the face'. At the same time I am disciplined about daily exercise to keep my muscles tight, my bones strong and my mental acuity pumped up with oxygen and those wonderful endorphins. Every woman is different, but for me, the daily ritual that keeps the motor purring is to down a dollop of Royal Jelly on awakening, to use nothing but natural oils on my face, and to bounce off (with the beat of fifties rock oldies plugged into my ear) to take a jog on nice days or work out with free weights and a treadmill. If time is short, I jump up and down on a tiny portable trampoline. I try to balance these weight-bearing efforts that are so good for the bones with meditation or a yoga class; it puts some elasticity back into sore sinews and stops the beat of urban life long enough to allow one to centre.

Like many women who found motherhood deeply satisfying, I now find myself drawn irresistibly to gardening. Whether it's planting pots of petunias on a balcony or digging a fragrant herb garden, perhaps pitching earth and nurturing tender blooms is our subjective way of replacing the joy of growing babies. I plant a new tree each year and take pleasure in watching its progress like a child moving through school. And whenever I'm in London, I look for offbeat bulbs for my Shakespeare garden; they never fail to amaze and delight me when they finally sprout.

Vitamins are vital at this age – C, E, B$_6$, and of course calcium enriched with Vitamin D. Since natural sources of calcium are best, I take milk on my cereal and in my coffee, and often a glass of warm skimmed milk at night to put me to sleep. Annual mammograms and biannual bone density checks are part of my discipline. Happily, I have *built* bone since I turned fifty with this regimen of exercise and hormone replacement. Finally, for husbanding my energy (and energizing my husband) I find that getting away together every six weeks or so for a long weekend adds immeasurably to the sweetness of life. And with our children grown, we can take off at the drop of a hat!

It has been a long road, but having 'rounded the horn' I feel rekindled, high-spirited and at home again inside my body. According to my husband, I look better, even younger, than I did when the journey began. (Thank goodness for the near-sightedness of middle age!) I am not the same me any more. I am an older woman, that is true. The energy is not the same jumpy fits-and-starts sort I had as a younger woman; it is deeper, sustained, and with naps for refreshment, it seldom fails me. The outlines of my future self are coming into focus – and I like her. She is focused but not so driven. She dares me to follow my purest instincts in what I think and read and write, rather than what is expected or externally valued. Do serious work and try to make a difference in the world, yes. But she won't let me neglect that part of myself that wants to play, that is rediscovering the harmless things I did as a young girl – like getting lost in the woods. She dares me to take off on adventures. I've decided I'll go along on the trip with her, believing that the best stages are yet to be.

The magic charm, finally, is very simple. It is to say to yourself, *No, I won't go back. And I won't try to stay in the same place, inside the same skin. I will go forward. I feel I will have the courage to take the next step.*

I believe it is vital to develop a future self in the mind's eye. She is our better nature, with bits and pieces of the most vital mature women we have known or read about and wish to emulate. If we are going to go grey, or white, we can pick out the most elegant white-haired woman we know and incorporate that element into our own inner picture. The more clearly we visualize our ideal future self, admire her indomitable skeleton and the grooves of experience that make up the map of her face, the more comfortable we will be with moving into her container.

An inspiring public model of wisewoman power is Elizabeth Cady Stanton. As one who pursued justice for women well into her eighties, Stanton was living proof of her belief which was eloquently recounted in her autobiography:

'The heyday of a woman's life is the shady side of fifty, when the vital forces heretofore expended in other ways are garnered in the brain, when their thoughts and sentiments flow out in broader channels, when philanthropy takes the place of family selfishness, and when from the depths of poverty and suffering the wail of humanity grows as pathetic to their ears as once was the cry of their own children.'

Today's 'coalescents' – both men and women – are mapping out a whole new stage of life for which evolution never provided. And we bring to it a broader view of the world. The source of continuing aliveness is to find your passion, and pursue it. It is essential to *claim the pause*. Remember, if forty-five is the old age of youth, fifty is the youth of a woman's Second Adulthood.

We are all pilgrims together, finding our way, but the markers we lay along the trail will beckon future generations to even longer lives. Filled with new life and licence, let us mark the way well.

Index

Index

My Mother/My Self

Nancy Friday

Why are women the way they are? Why, despite, everything, do we find so much of ourselves mysterious? Where do the dependence, the longing for intimacy, the passivity come from?

Drawing on her own and other women's lives, Nancy Friday shows compellingly that the key lies in a woman's relationship with her mother – that first binding relationship which becomes the model for so much of our adult relationships with men, and whose fetters constrain our sexuality, our independence, our very selfhood.

'Brilliant. Courageous. Moving. One of the most important books I have ever read about my mother, myself and my life.'

Washington Post

'A book most women will want to read and every man ought to.' Michael Korda

Jealousy

Nancy Friday

Why do so many intelligent, successful women get trapped in relationships where they are miserable, insecure and jealous? Why is jealousy so often the hook that keeps us in a relationship we would otherwise have left months before? Why do women's feelings about their best female friends so often include envy? And why do most men deny they ever feel jealous?

This crucial, unputdownable book, the result of a four-year personal quest, throws light on to every area of human relationships.

Toxic Psychiatry

Drugs and Electro-Convulsive Therapy: The Truth and the Better Alternatives

Peter Breggin

With an introduction and notes by Dorothy Rowe

'This book should create a sensation – let's hope it also helps to get people of toxic drugs.' Kate Millet, author of *The Loony-Bin Trip*

Are you or people you know being given any of these drugs?
Prozac, Xanax, Valium, Buspar, Ativan, Klonopin, Elavil, Tofranil, Haldol, Mellaril, Prolixin, Navane, Clozaril, Lithium, Ritalin.

There is no evidence to support the claims of the medical-pharmaceutical establishment that mental illnesses – such as schizophrenia, depression, manic-depression, panic disorder, obsessive-compulsive disorder or attention deficit disorder – are physical or genetic and can be cured by drugs or ECT. The truth is that, while these treatments justify the existence of, and fund, the industry, millions of people – school-children, housewives, the elderly, victims of childhood abuse, 'problem adolescents' and so on – are not being told that the 'miracle' cures they are being prescribed can cause serious brain damage.

In this groundbreaking book, psychiatrist Peter Breggin exposes in minute scientfic detail, and with carefully documented evidence, exactly what the horrifying effects are that the patients of psychiatry are not being informed about, and goes on to describe the resounding success he has experienced with more human alternatives for the treatment of mental illness – talking therapy, guidance, family therapy, rehabilitation and the teaching of coping skills – over the last twenty years.

'This has been one of the great reading experiences of my life . . . an all-out attack against the deception, half-truths and downright lies of psychiatry.' Jeffrey Mason, author of *Against Therapy*, *The Assault on Truth*, and *Final Analysis*

Fontana

Love Isn't Quite Enough
The Psychology of Male–Female Relationships

Maryon Tysoe

Finding out that love isn't quite enough is something most men and women do the hard way.

The traditional Western myth of romantic love has much to answer for. Both sexes can be devastated when they discover that, far from having the power of a psychological superglue, love is only one of many elements needed to sustain a relationship. Even those who are aware of – or reluctantly suspect – this are left floundering as to what other mysterious processes might be involved.

In *Love Isn't Quite Enough*, Dr Maryon Tysoe, widely admired social psychologist and journalist, has written an indispensable book for those seeking a better understanding of how relationships really work, why they fail and what we need to know to make them succeed. With characteristic wit and insight, she draws on a great deal of untapped psychological research to explore the route towards more realistic, and hence potentially more successful, relationships between the sexes.

'A wise, witty and highly readable book'   Dr Anthony Clare

Fontana

The Successful Self
Freeing our Hidden Inner Strengths

Dorothy Rowe

Is it possible to be truly successful as a person? Or must we, as most of us do, continue to live our lives feeling in some way trapped and oppressed, frustrated, irritable, haunted by worries and regrets, creating misery for ourselves and others?

In *The Successful Self* leading psychologist Dorothy Rowe, author of *Beyond Fear*, shows us how to live more comfortably and creatively within ourselves by achieving a fuller understanding of how we experience our existence and how we perceive the threat of its annihilation.

She demonstrates how to develop the social and personal skills we lack, retaining the uniqueness of our individuality while becoming an integral part of the life around us and learning how to value and accept ourselves.

With haracteristic originality, clarity and unfailing wisdom, Dorothy Rowe enables us to revolutionise our own lives and the lives of others in the process of becoming a Successful Self.

'Dorothy Rowe stands out amongst psychologists for her clear insight into human experience: her writing is refreshingly free from the dubious theoretical constructs and jargon ideas which plague this subject.'
Oliver Gillie, *Independent*

'A very brightly written book that intriguingly makes you question something most of us discuss: do we really like ourselves? Then it goes on to help us do so.' Mavis Nicholson

Choosing Not Losing

The Experiences of Depression

Dorothy Rowe

'I remember feeling very isolated. For a while I became convinced that I was set apart. Everyone seemed so well and confident. I marvelled that they were able to get through the day.'

Depression is the greatest isolation we can experience, a prison which we build for ourselves. Just as we build it, however, so we can unlock the door and let ourselves out.

In *Choosing Not Losing*, eminent psychologist Dorothy Rowe draws on her experiences with a number of patients who were referred to her for treatment. Their stories show that the lives of even those in the depths of depression can change.

A sympathetic and immensely valuable book, full of insight into the often strange and moving world of suffering inhabited by the depressive, *Choosing Not Losing* will give hope to all who read it.